What People Are Saying About *Cooking*

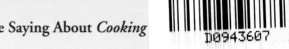

"When I was first placed on a gluten-free diet, I was lost as to how to survive in this gluten-filled world. Your cookbook provided much-needed guidance for cooking, baking, and eating well—gluten free."

—Peggy Wagener, Publisher, *Living Without,* a lifestyle guide for people with allergies and food sensitivities

"After working as a nutritionist for twenty years, I have found no allergy cookbook that compares to this wonderful reference. It contains the *best*-tasting recipes you will ever find!"

—Ellen Speare, B.S., Nutritionist

"A normal cookbook for special people."

—Ann Whelan, Publisher, *Gluten-Free Living* magazine

"Well written, informative, appealing, unique."

—Sheila E. Crowe, M.D., Associate Professor, Department of Internal Medicine, University of Virginia

"I like the idea of targeting dietary needs for special occasions."

—Joanne M. Vitanza, M.D., formerly of Colorado Allergy and Asthma Centers, P.C.

"A great source of information. Much needed by our patients."

—Dianna S. Hayton, R.N., Patient Educator, Colorado Allergy and Asthma Centers, P.C.

"You offer extra 'tidbits' that ensure success. A personal invitation to cooking success."

—Nancy Carol Sanker, OTR, former Education and Support Group Project Director, Asthma and Allergy Foundation of America

COOKING FREE

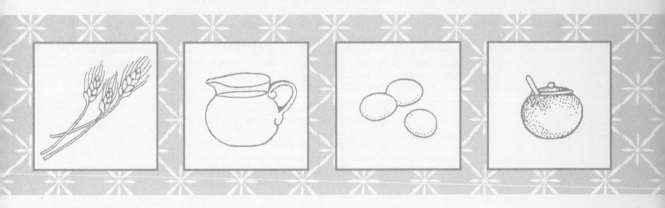

200 Flavorful Recipes for People with Food Allergies

and Multiple Food Sensitivities

CAROL FENSTER, PH.D.

Revised and updated recipes from *Special Diet Solutions* and *Special Diet Celebrations*

Avery

a member of Penguin Group (USA) Inc.

New York

Published by the Penguin Group

Penguin Group (USA) Inc., 375 Hudson Street, New York, New York 10014, USA • Penguin Group (Canada), 90 Eglinton Avenue East, Suite 700, Toronto, Ontario M4P 2Y3, Canada (a division of Pearson Penguin Canada Inc.) • Penguin Books Ltd, 80 Strand, London WC2R 0RL, England • Penguin Ireland, 25 St Stephen's Green, Dublin 2, Ireland (a division of Penguin Books Ltd) • Penguin Group (Australia), 250 Camberwell Road, Camberwell, Victoria 3124, Australia (a division of Pearson Australia Group Pty Ltd) • Penguin Books India Pvt Ltd, 11 Community Centre, Panchsheel Park, New Delhi–110 017, India • Penguin Group (NZ), Cnr Airborne and Rosedale Roads, Albany, Auckland 1310, New Zealand (a division of Pearson New Zealand Ltd) • Penguin Books (South Africa) (Pty) Ltd, 24 Sturdee Avenue, Rosebank, Johannesburg 2196, South Africa

Penguin Books Ltd, Registered Offices:
80 Strand, London WC2R 0RL, England

Library of Congress Cataloging-in-Publication Data

Fenster, Carol Lee.
Cooking free: 200 flavorful recipes for people with food allergies and multiple food sensitivities / Carol Fenster.
p. cm.
Includes bibliographical references and index.
ISBN 1-58333-215-4
1. Food allergy—Diet therapy—Recipes. I. Title.
RC588.D53F46   2005   2005041210
641.5'631—dc22

Printed in the United States of America
3 5 7 9 10 8 6 4 2

Book design by Meighan Cavanaugh

Neither the author nor the publisher is engaged in rendering professional advice or services to the individual reader. The ideas, procedures, and suggestions in this book are not intended as a substitute for consulting a physician. All matters regarding health require medical supervision. Neither the author nor the publisher shall be liable or responsible for any loss, injury, or damage allegedly arising from any information or suggestion in this book. The opinions expressed in this book represent the personal views of the author and not of the publisher.

The recipes contained in this book are to be followed exactly as written. Neither the publisher nor the author is responsible for your specific health or allergy needs that may require medical supervision, or for any adverse reactions to the recipes contained in this book.

While the author has made every effort to provide accurate telephone numbers and Internet addresses at the time of publication, neither the publisher nor the author assumes any responsibility for errors or for changes that occur after publication.

Most Avery books are available at special quantity discounts for bulk purchase for sales promotions, premiums, fund-raising, and educational needs. Special books or book excerpts also can be created to fit specific needs. For details, write Penguin Group (USA) Inc. Special Markets, 375 Hudson Street, New York, NY 10014.

To Larry, Brett, Helke, and Keene,
and in loving memory of Jeanne Von Wyl

ACKNOWLEDGMENTS

Food is usually the centerpiece of any social gathering. This cookbook was a joy to write because I know it will be used to make the food served appropriate for everyone with food sensitivities. I am deeply indebted to the following people who gave so generously of their time so you could safely take part in these gatherings.

To those who helped with testing recipes and providing excellent feedback, I truly appreciate your input—and please extend my thanks to your family and friends who lent their taste buds to the tasting process: Jane Dennison-Bauer; Julie Cary; Mary Courtney; Sandy Dempsey; Terri Ditmer; Laura Dolson; Donna Franz; Caroline Herdle; Jane Holcomb; Ruth Horelica; Janene Lenard; Alicia Pitzer; Janet Rinehart; Denise Roth; Lynn Samuel, LPN; Judy Sarver; Chris Silker; Jenny View; Peggy Wagener; Anne Washburn; Cecile Weed; and Sue Weilgopolan.

To those who helped with reviewing the manuscript and providing extremely valuable feedback, I sincerely appreciate your help: Rosanne G. Ainscough, R.D., CDE, Diabetes Dietitian Educator; Mary Bonner, Technical Writer; Gail Bright, R.D., Colorado Allergy and Asthma Centers; Sheila E. Crowe, M.D., Department of Internal Medicine, University of Virginia; Kathy Gibbons, Ph.D., Healthy Actions; Leon Greos, M.D., Colorado Allergy and Asthma Centers, P.C.; Dianna S. Hayton, R.N., Patient Educator, Colorado Allergy and Asthma Centers, P.C.; Cynthia Kupper, R.D., Executive Director, Gluten Intolerance Group; Anne Munoz-Furlong, Founder, Food Allergy & Anaphylaxis Network; Janet Y. Rinehart, Chairman, Houston Celiac Sprue Support Group and Past President, CSA/USA, Inc.; Nancy Carol Sanker, OTR, former Education and Support Group Project Director, Asthma and Allergy Foundation of America; Ellen Speare, B.S., Clinical Nutritionist, formerly of Wild Oats Markets; Gail Spiegel, M.S., R.D., CDE; Joanne M. Vitanza, M.D., formerly of Colorado Allergy and Asthma Centers, P.C.; Peggy A. Wagener, publisher of *Living Without* magazine; Ann Whelan, publisher of *Gluten-Free Living* newsletter; and Maura Zazenski.

I am enormously grateful to Lisa Ekus, my wonderful, inspiring agent, for her guidance, support, and unflagging enthusiasm for my work. I want to thank John Duff, Rebecca Behan, and especially my editor, Kristen Jennings, at Avery for their invaluable feedback on the book at various stages of the way.

Finally, a very special thank-you to my family—husband, Larry; son, Brett; daughter-in-law, Helke; and grandson, Keene. I love you all.

CONTENTS

Ingredients & Condiments

106

※

Main Dishes

121

※

Desserts

169

PREFACE

Managing a healthy diet can be challenging for anyone, but it's all the more so when common ingredients like wheat, dairy, eggs, and cane sugar must be avoided because of food sensitivities, medical conditions, and other special diet needs. For the 11 million Americans with some sort of reaction to food, even a simple meal with family and friends can be downright dangerous.

In addition to being a culinary professional, I am a sociologist who is fascinated by the symbolism of food. Rituals associated with food—even if just nightly suppers around the kitchen table—become the memories of a lifetime. And yet for those of us with food sensitivities, dining on any occasion can be risky. Even food we once ate—and that everyone expects us to continue eating—is now off-limits. But the good news is that you can continue to eat these foods—if they're prepared with appropriate substitutes for the problem ingredients. Fortunately, my training as a home economist and my own personal struggle with gluten intolerance have given me the technical ability to transform recipes into dishes that everyone can safely enjoy.

If you've read my first book, *Wheat-Free Recipes & Menus: Delicious, Healthful Eating for People with Food Sensitivities* (Avery, 2004), you know my story. I suffered from chronic sinusitis for decades until I learned to avoid my own particular food villains—wheat and wheat-related grains. For someone raised on a farm in Nebraska and who married into a wheat-farming family—complete with a father-in-law who is an internationally recognized expert on wheat cultivation—this was unsettling, to say the least.

The irony is that wheat caused my lifetime struggle with nasal congestion and stuffiness—making me feel dull, groggy, and lethargic. For decades, I was plagued by chronic sinus infections requiring endless rounds of antibiotics. It always seemed like I was "coming down with a cold," and my sinus infections were often accompanied by laryngitis and bronchitis. And my eighty-hour workweek as a corporate marketing executive—interspersed with far too much transcontinental travel—didn't help.

I never suspected wheat as the culprit. I didn't understand that the proteins in wheat—particularly gluten—can be toxic to many of us. I didn't associate my fondness for baked goods—bagels, fresh-baked bread, pasta, cakes, and cookies—with the chronic congestion. And I had no idea that wheat lurked in the most unsuspecting places, such as licorice candy. Or that wheat is actually related to barley, rye, spelt, and kamut—which also must be avoided.

It took several decades for me to discover that wheat is my nemesis and that I'm part of the 10 to 15 percent of Americans who can't eat it. In fact, when I was diagnosed I kept hoping the doctor was wrong and that he would eventually call me to say it was all a big mistake. To make matters worse, I didn't know anyone else who couldn't eat wheat, so I felt isolated. And, of course, my new wheat-free way of life was puzzling to my wheat-farming family.

After my diagnosis, I knew I had to take complete control over what I ate if I wanted to regain my health. So I began researching how I could prepare the same dishes I was accustomed to eating, while eliminating wheat as an ingredient. I learned which alternative flours were acceptable to my diet and how these flours perform in various recipes. Eventually I totally revamped my family's repertoire of dishes, and after a great deal of what my daughter-in-law calls "dishes, discourse, and discovery," I mastered the gluten-free lifestyle. I decided to turn my recipes into a cookbook and founded my company, Savory Palate, Inc., with the mission of helping others eat well without gluten.

However, when I began teaching gluten-free cooking classes at local health food stores, I learned that wheat wasn't the only food culprit. Many students told me that they couldn't eat dairy products, or that eggs bothered them, or that cane sugar was on their forbidden list. From them, the idea for this book was born.

I compiled everything I learned into this book, which is not only wheat-free but also includes recipes so versatile that they can be used by individuals or families with a variety of *other* food sensitivities—particularly to dairy, eggs, and cane sugar—and no one will feel deprived. Believe me, it took a lot more sessions of dishes, discourse, and discovery in my kitchen to figure out how to cook foods free of the most common food allergens. Although the recipes don't offer specific substitutes for corn or soy, you can also avoid these ingredients if you're careful to read ingredient labels and find replacements.

Today—after all this kitchen testing and learning—I am an expert in helping people with special diet needs manage a healthy regimen. Once they identify their own particular food villains with the assistance of a health professional, I help them eat the foods they love—without the ingredients they don't want. There is almost always an appropriate substitute for a particular ingredient. The secret lies in knowing what the substitute is and how to use it. I've created this cookbook so you will know *exactly* what to do.

You'll notice I don't refer to the foods in this book as being part of a restricted, limited, or alternative diet. Instead, I refer to them as part of a "special" diet, because it is tailored to suit the needs of those with food allergies. I'm aware of the psychological aspects of adjusting to this way of eating in terms of the grief, denial, and anger that accompany loss of any kind, including that of some of your favorite foods. However, it is important to refer to your diet with a positive, rather than negative, outlook. Our bodies hear what our brains are thinking, so keep your thoughts and actions positive at all times. To me, "special" is a positive term. Whenever I'm tempted by forbidden food, I say to myself, "Nothing tastes as good as feeling good feels." I then imagine how I will feel if I eat the forbidden food—that's enough to make me realize it isn't worth it.

Some people love to cook. However, many others tell me they don't like to cook, don't have time to prepare meals, or feel inadequate in the kitchen. Despite the growing availability of mixes and ready-made foods, you will need to prepare some dishes yourself. Yes, this usually requires preparing most dishes from scratch. But, it's important to remain positive. There are three major benefits when you cook from scratch: (1) you gain control over what you eat, (2) you control the standards under which that food is prepared, and (3) you can enjoy the physiological aspects of seeing, touching, smelling, and, yes, hearing your food (think of bacon sizzling in a hot skillet). Nothing beats creating a tasty dish that you, your family, and your guests enjoy. Who knows, you may actually start to look forward to your time in the kitchen, especially if you can talk other family members into helping you with the food preparation.

A lot has changed since I wrote my first cookbook in 1995. Back then, the wheat-free diet was considered unusual. One well-meaning allergist told me that my first book would be a "labor of love" and nothing more because there were so few wheat-free patients. Celiac disease—a particular form of wheat sensitivity in which gluten, a protein in wheat, damages the digestive system—was virtually unknown to the general public. The medical community didn't pay much attention to celiac disease, labeling it a "rare" condition. Mainstream manufacturers, restaurants, and other businesses in the food industry barely acknowledged the wheat-free diet, leaving it to a handful of specialized entrepreneurs to fill the void with cookbooks, mixes, and a few ready-made foods.

Today, the focus on wheat sensitivity has been expanded to include wheat's cousins barley, rye, and spelt—all of which contain gluten, the major offender. So, we now call it the gluten-free diet. Leading universities, such as the University of Maryland, Columbia, Stanford, University of Chicago, and the University of Southern California, have established celiac research centers. Restaurants offer gluten-free dishes, new gluten-free foods appear on grocery shelves or are available from an extensive array of online vendors, and in August 2003, NBC's *Today* show featured a segment on celiac disease.

Specialized magazines, such as *Gluten-Free Living,* carefully research which ingredients are gluten-free and which aren't. Another magazine, *Living Without,* offers gluten-free advice plus recipes and lifestyle articles for people with various types of food sensitivities. My cookbooks have been joined by others, so that we all have choices when we cook at home.

In 2003, leaders in the gluten-free community formed the American Celiac Task Force to present a unified voice to government, the food industry, and the public at www.celiaccenter.org/taskforce.asp. In June 2004, the National Institutes of Health (NIH) Consensus Development Conference on Celiac Disease defined celiac disease, its diagnosis, and treatment.

At the same time that the gluten-free diet was gaining acceptance, other food allergens were also being addressed on Capitol Hill. During the summer of 2004, the Food Allergen Labeling and Consumer Protection Act was passed, mandating that by 2006 food manufacturers will be required to label products if they contain any of these top eight allergens: wheat, dairy, eggs, soy, fish, shellfish, tree nuts, or peanuts. All of this means that there will be greater attention to the allergens addressed in this book. If there were ever a time to have a food sensitivity—it's now.

INTRODUCTION

As surprising as it may seem, any food can be an allergen for any person (although I must confess that I've never heard of anyone being allergic to rutabaga). However, eight foods produce 90 percent of the food reactions in America: wheat, dairy, eggs, soy, fish, shellfish, tree nuts, and peanuts. Of those, wheat, dairy, and eggs—along with cane sugar—make up some of the most common ingredients in foods and can be the most difficult for those with intolerances to avoid. In this book, you will find creative ways to make delicious meals without these common allergens so that you can stay healthy while eating well.

According to the Food Allergy & Anaphylaxis Network (FAAN), about 11 million Americans suffer from food allergies. True food allergies—as opposed to less severe intolerances—involve the immune system, and reactions are usually sudden and pronounced. For example, I know of a young man who is so allergic to wheat that he had an anaphylactic reaction after entering a kitchen while somebody was baking. He apparently ingested some wheat flour particles that were floating through the air and was rushed to the emergency room for treatment, after using his Epi-Pen to buy him more time. Few people have food allergies this severe, but for those who do, rigid restrictions and lifestyle changes must be adhered to.

Compared to the relatively few people with true food allergies, far more people—estimates are as high as 25 percent of all Americans—have food intolerances. In contrast to food allergies, reactions involved in food intolerances *may* be delayed and are usually subtler.

My reaction to gluten, for example, is classified as an intolerance. Those like me experience nasal congestion and stuffiness, a feeling of fatigue, and what we affectionately call "brain fog." In my case, nasal stuffiness might be faintly apparent by the end of a wheat-laden meal yet become full-blown congestion by the next morning and be accompanied by overwhelming fatigue and a definite "fogginess." However, the reactions associated with food intolerances can take many different forms, including headaches (sometimes migraines), stomachaches, rashes, achy joints, and a host of other maladies that are as easily associated with other ailments, often making it difficult to pinpoint food intolerances. These same types of reactions may occur with other foods such as dairy and eggs, as well. Food intolerances won't kill you, but they certainly compromise the quality of your life. Furthermore, the treatment for the symptoms can be as devastating as the symptoms themselves. In my case, endless rounds of antibiotics have had a profound and lasting effect on my digestive system by making me more sensitive to yeast and molds.

Diagnosis of a food allergy or intolerance should be made by a board-certified allergist or a health professional who specializes in this area. There are a variety of tests and procedures used to confirm a diagnosis. Testing for food allergies and intolerances remains a somewhat controversial area, and not all experts agree on a single approach. For more information on food allergies and intolerances, refer to the resources in the back of the book, including the listings for the Food Allergy & Anaphylaxis Network and York Nutritional Laboratories.

Whether you are truly allergic or intolerant, you need to know how to cook without problem ingredients. Ordinarily, wheat is a nutritious food, and its marvelous baking properties make it our country's grain of choice. Milk, eggs, and sugar also play important roles in baking. There are many reasons why the ingredients eliminated from the recipes in this book—wheat, dairy, eggs, and cane sugar—may not be appropriate for everyone. Each of you reading this right now has a unique story, but basically most of you will be sensitive to one or more of the following types of foods.

GLUTEN

Gluten is a protein found in wheat and related grains such as barley, rye, spelt, kamut, and triticale. Some people can be allergic to gluten, while others (like me) are gluten intolerant. Celiac disease is different from allergies and intolerances in that it is an auto-immune reaction to gluten. There are many other medical conditions that require individuals to avoid gluten. For example, part of the treatment for various autoimmune conditions such as multiple sclerosis, rheumatoid arthritis, and lupus may include a gluten-free diet. Persons with autism and food-triggered asthma are also sometimes placed on gluten-free diets. You should rely on the advice of your physician as to whether a gluten-free diet is appropriate for you. But, if it is, this book will help you.

All of the recipes in this book avoid wheat and any wheat-related grains such as barley, rye, spelt, or kamut by using gluten-free flours and by specifying gluten-free substitutes for other ingredients as well. They also avoid oats (see discussion below). Each recipe is gluten-free, but occasionally you will need to make sure you select a gluten-free version of a particular ingredient. For example, some brands of chicken broth contain wheat, but gluten-free versions exist. The gluten-free icon in front of the ingredient means you must find a gluten-free brand of chicken broth.

CELIAC DISEASE

Celiac disease is an inherited autoimmune disorder that affects the digestive process in the small intestine. When a person who has celiac disease consumes gluten—a protein found in wheat, rye, barley, spelt, kamut, and triticale—the individual's immune system responds by attacking the small intestine and inhibiting the absorption of important nutrients into the body. Undiagnosed and untreated, celiac disease can lead to the development of other disorders, such as osteoporosis, infertility, neurological conditions, and, in rare cases, cancer. Another form of the disease called dermatitis herpetiformis (DH) includes symptoms such as skin rashes and blisterlike spots.

Celiac disease is far more common than originally thought. Once deemed extremely rare, celiac disease affects 1 in 133 people—or nearly 3 million people—in the United States, according to the National Institutes of Health Consensus Development Conference on Celiac Disease, June 2004. Interestingly, this condition is much more common than many other diseases that get far more attention. For example, according to the University of Chicago Celiac Disease Program (quoting from the National Institutes of Health), celiac disease affects more people than those with Parkinson's disease (500,000), or rheumatoid arthritis (2.1 million) or multiple sclerosis (333,000). Unlike these other diseases, however, there is no pill, no vaccine, and no surgical procedure. The only treatment is a gluten-free diet for life. Even in persons who don't exhibit the typical symptoms (diarrhea, bloating, gas, or fatigue), damage to the intestines can still occur if gluten is ingested.

Those with celiac disease must avoid *all* forms of gluten, which is present in wheat and wheat-related grains such as barley, rye, spelt, possibly oats, and the lesser-known grains of kamut and triticale. Gluten also lurks in many innocent-looking commercial foods, so careful reading of labels is very important.

Unfortunately, despite its prevalence, celiac disease takes an average of eleven years to diagnose. It must be managed with the help of a gastroenterologist, who performs a series of tests—including a small bowel endoscopy while the patient is sedated—before a final diagnosis can be made. For more information on celiac disease, see the Resources section in the back of the book.

AUTISM—A SPECIAL INTOLERANCE

Approximately 1 in 160 children is estimated to have autism, a number that seems to be rising. A serious neurobiological disorder, autism perplexes adults and the medical community alike. As part of the overall treatment (but not as a substitute for other treatment), several experts advocate a gluten-free, casein-free diet (casein is a milk protein). Apparently, some autistic children don't process these proteins properly and removing the proteins from these children's diet helps their behavior.

For more information on autism and the gluten-free, casein-free diet, consult your physician. Several associations, included in the Resources section, provide information about autism. You'll find more specific information on the diet at www.gfcfdiet.com.

WHAT IT MEANS TO LIVE ON
A GLUTEN-FREE DIET

You may have noticed that I use both terms, "wheat-free" and "gluten-free." Technically, wheat-free implies that you avoid only wheat while continuing to eat wheat's cousins barley, rye, and spelt. However, this book is gluten-free, meaning that there is no gluten of any kind—wheat, any of its cousins, or oats—in any of the recipes (remember, gluten is the protein in wheat that causes us so much trouble). So, for the remainder of this book, I'll use the term "gluten-free."

So, what does living gluten-free mean? It means being aware of everything you put in your mouth. You need to query chefs and servers in restaurants while being polite but firm when someone insists that you should eat something you know will make you sick. Awareness of everything you eat means you must know exactly what's in your food. This means reading labels and understanding the meaning of the words on the ingredients list. For more information on hidden gluten, see Common Sources of Wheat and Gluten in Appendix B.

One particularly helpful source is the *Quick Start Diet Guide,* jointly published by the Gluten Intolerance Group of North America and the Celiac Disease Foundation, which outlines the dos and don'ts of the gluten-free diet in simple, easy-to-understand terms. It can be a bit daunting to keep up with which ingredients are safe and which aren't. Some associations provide lists of commercial products that are known to be safe. You can order the Commercial Product Listing from the Celiac Sprue Association (877-CSA-4-CSA), or the Tri-Counties shopping list from Tri-County Celiac Sprue Group. In addition, *Gluten-Free Living* magazine (www.glutenfreeliving.com) reviews the safety of various ingredients. See the Resources section for access to these and other helpful guides.

A few foods—oats, liquor, vinegar, and vanilla—continue to generate questions. Here is a brief discussion on the latest knowledge about these issues, gleaned primarily from *Gluten-Free Living* magazine. With helpful sources like these, you gradually learn the ropes, and the diet becomes a way of life. I've been *totally* gluten-free for more than ten years now and I know that I eat a much healthier diet—more fresh fruits and vegetables, less processed meat, and fewer refined foods.

OATS—THE CURRENT STATUS

Oats have traditionally been excluded from the gluten-free diet even though experts agree that oats do not inherently contain gluten. The explanation is that oats *may* be contaminated with wheat because the two crops are grown in the same field during consecutive years (called rotation) and because their remarkably similar-looking kernels can be intermingled in manufacturing.

Several studies show that oats are safe to eat on a gluten-free diet—at least on a short-term basis. But experts are reluctant to encourage eating oats on a regular basis because there are no studies documenting the long-term effects of oat consumption. Nor are any manufacturers willing to guarantee their oats as gluten-free. To be on the safe side, I don't use oats in any recipe in this book and I don't recommend them to anyone on a gluten-free diet. Check with your physician about eating oats.

DISTILLED SPIRITS, VINEGAR, AND VANILLA

Except for wine, gin, and tequila, alcoholic beverages have traditionally been omitted from the gluten-free diet. However, a careful review by *Gluten-Free Living* magazine of the process by which distilled spirits are made shows that scotch, whiskey, bourbon, and other distilled spirits are safe because the gluten peptides cannot survive the distillation process. Of course, any alcoholic beverage that is made from gluten-containing grains and that is not distilled—such as beer—still contains gluten.

Vinegar is another ingredient that has traditionally been suspect. However, even if vinegar is made with gluten-containing grains (which it probably isn't, because vinegar is usually made from corn), the gluten in these grains cannot survive the distillation process. The same is true of vanilla extract. This means you can use regular vanilla (instead of alcohol-free) and enjoy salad dressings made with vinegar—unless, of course, vanilla or vinegar bothers you for other reasons. For example, some people have sensitivities to fermented foods. If so, you should avoid them.

If you are on a gluten-free diet, you *must* avoid malt vinegar, though. It contains gluten because the malt is added back in *after* the distillation process, using barley for the flavoring. (For a thorough discussion of distilled spirits, vanilla, and vinegar, see *Gluten-Free Living* magazine, Sept./Oct. and Nov./Dec. 1999 and Vol. 8, #3, 2003.)

DAIRY

According to the National Institutes of Health (NIH), as many as 30 to 50 million Americans are lactose intolerant. Lactose intolerance occurs when the body lacks lactase, an enzyme needed to digest the milk sugar called lactose. The condition affects some ethnic groups more than others: as many as 75 percent of African-Americans and 90 percent of Asian-Americans are lactose intolerant.

People can also be allergic to dairy products. There aren't official statistics on the exact number of milk-allergic persons, but the number is far smaller than those with lactose intolerance because the overall incidence of food allergies in general is around 3 percent of all Americans. There are several proteins in milk, but it is usually the milk proteins casein and whey that cause the most trouble.

Since lactose intolerance is one of the most common food sensitivities in America, and the ability of many celiacs to digest lactose is impaired (especially during the early healing stages), I offer suggestions for dairy substitutes for milk, butter, and cheese in all recipes except those that must be dairy-based to work properly. When you need to choose a dairy-free version of an ingredient, the recipe carries the dairy-free icon.

EGGS

It is the proteins in eggs that cause digestive reactions, although some people are truly allergic to eggs and others are intolerant to them. For most people, it is the egg whites that cause the reaction, while some react to the egg yolks. Most of the recipes in this book offer a safe substitute for eggs unless a particular recipe (such as Sally Lunn Bread) relies on eggs for leavening. In that case, the recipe will not carry the egg-free logo.

SUGAR

Sugar is a much-maligned food these days, particularly white sugar. This book is not designed for those who wish to avoid white sugar so they can reduce their caloric intake and lose weight. Instead, many people can't eat white sugar because they are sensitive to cane—the source of much of the white sugar used in America today. Some people can safely use beet sugar, the other major source of white sugar, but this doesn't work for everyone. Unfortunately, we don't have any official statistics on how many people are advised to avoid white sugar because of food sensitivities. For each recipe, I offer an alternative to the cane-based white or brown sugar. These recipes carry the sugar-free icon.

An extensive section in Appendix A, Baking with Alternative Sweeteners, offers a number of alternative sweeteners to white sugar or brown sugar and discusses how to use each sweetener to its best cooking or baking advantage. Almost all of these sweeteners have a caloric content similar to white sugar, although experts believe that some sweeteners are absorbed more slowly than others and thus have a less dramatic effect on blood sugar levels. Some sweeteners, such as agave nectar, have a low glycemic index (the rate at which the sugar is absorbed into the bloodstream).

It is beyond the scope of this book to analyze sweeteners from a glycemic index perspective, but for more information see *The New Glucose Revolution* by Jennie Brand-Miller, Thomas M.S. Wolever, Kaye Foster-Powell, and Stephen Colagiuri. The purpose of this book is to show you how to use alternative sweeteners—not to tell you if a particular sweetener is better for your blood sugar than another. By the way, you'll notice that I don't use any artificial sweeteners such as aspartame or saccharin. These sugar substitutes don't produce tasty baked goods when wheat, dairy, and eggs are omitted. You'll have to turn to other cookbooks for that information.

STOCKING THE
COOKING-FREE PANTRY

By now, you have realized some of the ingredients used in this book will be new to you. In addition to gluten-free flours, I recommend other ingredients that you may not have used before—or may not have used in the same ways as they are in these recipes—such as dry milk powder, egg replacer, and unflavored gelatin powder. Each plays a vital, sometimes critical, role in the success of allergen-free cooking. Stocking the Cooking-Free pantry is similar to stocking *any* pantry—but we use *different* ingredients in *our* pantry. In addition to the usual sugar, salt, pepper, and your favorite spices, basic ingredients you'll want to have on hand so you're prepared are listed on page 9. These ingredients are not necessarily in order of importance but are alphabetized instead. Beside each ingredient is a brief explanation of how you'll use it. Your pantry will expand as you discover other essential items. In addition to this list, I have provided a detailed Glossary of Ingredients in the back of the book (see page 296) so that you can find the definition and common uses of a broad range of ingredients you may not be familiar with.

THE IMPORTANCE OF READING FOOD LABELS

Reading labels is very important when shopping for foods to stock your Cooking-Free pantry. Learn to recognize the various names used for certain ingredients Also, *continue* to read labels on all ingredients—even the ones you've used for a long time. Manufacturers may change the contents of an ingredient, perhaps adding a substance. They may change the manner in which it was prepared, such as dusting the item with wheat flour to prevent sticking. Or the manufacturing process may introduce cross contamination with other problem ingredients. Call the manufacturer if you have concerns. Phrase your questions as clearly and concisely as possible and be sure to thank them for responding to your questions. See Appendix B for a list of foods and ingredients in which wheat, dairy, or eggs, may be hidden. I also offer a list of Common Sources of Corn and Common Sources of Soy for your reference, since these are two common allergens. However, none of the recipes in this book offers substitutes for corn or soy. You can avoid corn or soy by learning where these allergens are hidden in food and then avoid those foods.

INGREDIENT	ROLE
Baking powder, baking soda, cream of tartar	Leavening for baked goods.
Butter, shortening, margarine, cooking oil	Adds fat to baked goods; grease baking pans.
Dry milk powder (This is not Carnation instant milk granules. This is a fine powder, not granules.)	Adds protein, which improves the texture of bread, and provides food for yeast in baked goods.
Egg replacer powder (Ener-G Foods or Kingsmill)	Fine white powder that improves structure and texture of baked goods; adds leavening.
Flour: sorghum, rice, garbanzo/fava bean, corn, white bean, potato starch, cornstarch, tapioca, arrowroot, almond, chestnut, and sweet rice	Creates custom flour blends for baking; thickens sauces, gravies, and puddings.
Gelatin (unflavored) powder (Knox or Grayslake brand)	Adds moisture and protein to baked goods; binds ingredients together.
Lecithin granules: Made of soy, you can buy in supplement section of health food store.	Light-yellow granules that improve texture and emulsify (combine) ingredients by binding oil and water.
Pasta in all shapes/sizes (My favorite is penne.)	Use in casseroles, pasta dishes, soups.
Vinegar	"Sours" milk into buttermilk and is acidic food for yeast.
Xanthan gum, guar gum	Prevents crumbling in baked goods; thicken sauces and salad dressings. Either one or both are absolutely essential for successful gluten-free baking.
Yeast (Dry active; don't use rapid-rise yeast unless the recipe calls for it.)	Leavens baked goods and adds yeast flavor.

Cooking-Free Techniques

In addition to new ingredients, you'll find new techniques that seem to defy conventional kitchen wisdom—such as using an electric mixer to beat soft, sticky gluten-free dough rather than kneading it with your hands. Or putting bread dough into a *cold* oven instead of a preheated *hot* oven. Or mixing muffins with an electric mixer until they're well blended instead of the usual muffin method of adding liquid ingredients into the well of dry ingredients and stirring just until blended.

To cook with these sometimes unconventional cooking methods, you'll need the utensils and other apparatuses listed below. Again, these items are alphabetized rather than listed in order of importance.

APPLIANCES, UTENSILS, ETC.	PURPOSE
Nonstick (gray color, not black) loaf pans, baking sheets, pie pans, and cake pans	Prevents dough from sticking to pan. Gluten-free foods sometimes "stick," so nonstick pans are a must. Plus they brown food better than glass or shiny aluminum pans.
Parchment paper (silicone-lined paper)	Lines baking sheets for quick release of baked goods as well as easy cleanup.
Plastic wrap, foil, waxed paper, paper towels	Covers food; aids in handling and shaping dough and batter.
Stand mixer (I use a 4.5-qt. KitchenAid.)	Useful for beating heavy, gluten-free dough and batter.

Types of Recipes in This Book

Now that you know which food allergens are addressed in this book, you might like to know the types of recipes you can make. This is a comprehensive cookbook, meaning that it contains recipes for all the main categories of foods, including breads, breakfast and brunch, appetizers and snacks, salads and salad dressings, ingredients and condiments, main dishes, and desserts.

These recipes are perfect for any occasion, whether it's a weekday meal for your family or a special celebration. To help you with menu planning there are fourteen organized around certain types of meals ranging from simple to elegant, from picnics to dinner parties.

And, I haven't forgotten that children have food sensitivities too and need their own special kinds of food. For example, there are several recipes for basic cakes that you can decorate for a child's birthday party. There are also basic recipes for cookies that kids will not only love to eat but will also have fun decorating. And there is also a fabulous pizza recipe that kids of all ages love.

NUTRITIONAL CONTENT

Fortunately, the food allergen community is broadening its focus from concern only with safety ("Does it contain gluten or dairy?") to include a broader interest in nutrition as well. For example, today's consumers on a gluten-free diet want to know the nutrient content of their food, so all recipes in this book are analyzed using MasterCook software and provide information for each recipe on calories, fat, protein, carbohydrates, cholesterol, sodium, and fiber.

You'll find the nutrient content at the bottom of each recipe. These values are based on the United States Department of Agriculture (USDA) guidelines and are only approximate, since exact nutrient values may vary according to size of serving or particular brands of ingredients used.

Some of these nutrient values are rounded according to the Food and Drug Administration (FDA) guidelines. For example, if there are fewer than 5 grams of fat, the value is rounded to the nearest half gram. If there are more than 5 grams of fat, the value is rounded to the nearest whole number. Carbohydrates, proteins, sodium, and cholesterol are rounded to the nearest whole number. Calories are rounded to the nearest five calories. Fiber is rounded to the nearest half gram. When there is more than one choice of ingredients, the analysis is performed using the first ingredient listed.

Some consumers are also careful to include healthy fats, rather than hydrogenated versions, in their diets. So, my recipes use healthy oils such as canola or olive oil and require only the minimum amount needed to produce a tasty dish. In each recipe that uses margarine or shortening, a nonhydrogenated, trans fat–free substitute is suggested. Also, the nutritional analysis is based on using 2% milk.

SERVING SIZE

Serving sizes recommended by the American Diabetes Association are used in the calculation of nutrient values. Because we Americans are accustomed to eating very large portions, these serving sizes may seem quite small, and it may take several servings to satisfy you.

Family, friends, and good times are a central theme of this book. Many of us associate certain foods with special times in our lives. For me, it was a unique kind of cake that my mother made for my birthday party, or the special roasted chicken we shared with my aunts and cousins after long walks in the timberlands near our farm, or the dishes we ate at the neighborhood block parties when my son was growing up. I hope some of the recipes in this book will become your favorite dishes and that all of your family and friends will remember them in connection with good times.

AUTHOR'S NOTE

I wrote this cookbook as a resource for people on special diets—people who *know* they must avoid wheat or gluten and any (or all) of the other common food allergens, including dairy, eggs, and cane sugar. It is meant to help you eat the dishes you want after your health professional tells you which ingredients to avoid. This book should not be used to diagnose yourself or others, to determine whether you have a particular condition that warrants a special diet, or to determine the particular ingredients you should avoid. Let a health professional guide you in this process.

If you belong to any of the following groups of people, then the recipes in this book are appropriate for your diet:

1. People who *must* avoid gluten in their diets. This includes people with celiac disease (also known as celiac sprue, gluten intolerance, gluten sensitive enteropathy, and dermatitis herpetiformis). It also includes people with wheat allergies where even a little wheat can cause an anaphylactic reaction that could be fatal.
2. People who avoid wheat and all wheat-related grains because of gluten intolerances or other special dietary considerations such as autoimmune conditions (e.g., rheumatoid arthritis, multiple sclerosis, and lupus). This also includes autistic children who are sometimes placed on a gluten-free diet as part of their overall treatment plan.
3. Gluten-sensitive people who have *additional* sensitivities to dairy, eggs, and cane sugar.

BREADS

Hearty, flavorful breads complement any meal. They add wonderful flavor and help fill you up, and those crunchy crusts are fabulous. In fact, bread is what we miss the most on a gluten-free diet. But with the recipes here, you can indulge in the staff of life.

Many of you have asked for gluten-free breads that also contain no dairy or eggs. I'm happy to provide these bread recipes for you. Some are yeast leavened; others are quick breads that use baking soda or baking powder (or a combination of cream of tartar and baking soda).

My easy directions for each gluten-free recipe show you how to make the bread with or without eggs and milk—so you leave out only the ingredients you don't want. There are also bread-machine directions for loaf-shaped yeast breads. And you can choose to make some loaves in either 1- or 1½-pound sizes. Your family will love fresh-baked bread for dinner tonight, so start baking.

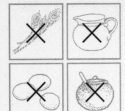

"CRACKED WHEAT" BREAD

Cracked brown rice imitates the texture of whole wheat in this bread. Crack the whole brown rice in a blender or coffee grinder until kernels are ¼ to ⅓ normal size.

	MAKES 1 POUND *Serves 12*	MAKES 2 POUNDS *Serves 18*
Active dry yeast	2¼ teaspoons	2¼ teaspoons
Brown sugar or maple sugar	1 tablespoon	2 tablespoons
Milk (cow, rice, or soy) (110°F)	1 cup	1½ cups
Flour Blend (page 276)	2½ cups	3⅓ cups
Whole brown rice, cracked	¼ cup	⅓ cup
Xanthan gum	1½ teaspoons	2 teaspoons
Salt	1 teaspoon	1½ teaspoons
Egg replacer powder	1 teaspoon	1½ teaspoons
Eggs or soft silken tofu	2 large eggs, or ½ cup soft silken tofu	3 large eggs, or ¾ cup soft silken tofu
Butter (melted) or oil	3 tablespoons	⅓ cup
Vinegar	1 teaspoon	2 teaspoons
Pans	Five 5x3-inch loaf pans, or one 9x5-inch loaf pan	Five 5x3-inch loaf pans, or two 8x4-inch loaf pans

HAND:

1. Combine yeast, brown sugar, and milk and set aside for 5 minutes. In large mixer bowl using electric beaters (not dough hooks), combine flours, rice, xanthan gum, salt, and egg replacer. In separate bowl, cream together eggs or tofu, butter, and vinegar until very smooth. With mixer on low, add egg mixture and yeast-milk mixture to dry ingredients and blend on high for 1 minute.

2. Generously grease loaf pans. Divide dough among prepared pans. Rise in warm place (75–80°F) until dough is level with top of pan.

3. Preheat oven to 350°F. Bake small loaves for 25–30 minutes, large loaves for 40–50 minutes, until tops are nicely browned. Cool for 5 minutes in pan. Remove from pan; cool on wire rack.

MACHINE:

Spray pan with cooking spray. Add room temperature ingredients in order listed by manufacturer. Set controls and bake.

Nutrition Information (per serving)

Calories 160 • Fat 5g • Protein 5g • Carbohydrates 26g • Cholesterol 41mg • Sodium 272mg • Fiber 1g

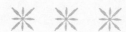

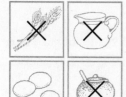

FRENCH BREAD

Makes 2 loaves (Serves 20, 1-inch slices)

Put this bread into a *cold* oven for a crisp crust and nice texture. If this doesn't work in your oven, let the bread rise until level with top of pan; then bake in preheated 425°F oven for 25–30 minutes. Use a pan specially designed for French bread.

1 tablespoon sugar or honey
2 tablespoons active dry yeast
1¼ cups warm water (110°F)
2 cups Flour Blend (page 276)
1 cup potato starch
1 teaspoon xanthan gum
1 teaspoon guar gum
¼ cup dry milk powder (cow, rice, or soy)

1½ teaspoons salt
1 tablespoon butter or margarine, softened
3 large egg whites
1 teaspoon vinegar
Egg white wash (optional—1 beaten egg white)

1. In bowl, dissolve sugar and yeast in warm water and set aside for 5 minutes.
2. Grease French bread pan or line with parchment paper.
3. In bowl of a heavy-duty stand mixer, combine remaining ingredients, except the egg wash, then add the yeast mixture. Beat on low speed to blend. Beat on high speed for 2 minutes, stirring down sides with spatula. Dough will be soft.
4. Divide dough in half on the prepared pan. Smooth each half into 12-inch-long log with wet spatula. Brush with egg wash for glossier crust, if desired. Make 3 diagonal slashes (⅛ inch deep) in each loaf so steam can escape during baking.
5. Place immediately on the middle rack of a *cold* oven. Set the temperature at 425°F and bake for 30–35 minutes, until nicely browned.
6. Remove bread from pan; cool completely on wire rack before slicing with electric knife.

Nutrition Information (per serving)
Calories 83 • Fat 1g • Protein 2g • Carbohydrates 17g • Cholesterol 2mg • Sodium 159mg • Fiber 0.5g

Variation

For garlic French bread, spread slices of French Bread with mixture of ½ cup softened butter or margarine and 1 garlic clove, minced. One tablespoon of butter adds 100 calories.

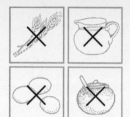

MULTIGRAIN SANDWICH BREAD

Makes a 1-pound loaf (Serves 12)

The addition of rice bran makes this versatile sandwich bread hearty and higher in fiber.

2 teaspoons active dry yeast

2 tablespoons granulated sugar or fructose powder, divided

1 cup warm milk (cow, rice, or soy) (110°F)

2 cups Flour Blend (page 276)

¼ cup rice bran

¼ cup finely chopped almonds or almond meal

2 teaspoons xanthan gum

1 teaspoon salt

¼ teaspoon potato flour (not potato starch)

2 large eggs, or ⅓ cup Flax Mix (page 108)

3 tablespoons canola oil

1 teaspoon vinegar

1. Grease 8x4-inch nonstick loaf pan. In bowl, combine yeast, 2 teaspoons of the sugar or fructose powder, and warm milk and set aside to let yeast foam, about 5 minutes.

2. In large bowl of heavy-duty tabletop mixer (300 watts or more) using beaters (not dough hooks), combine remaining ingredients, including remainder of sugar and yeast mixture.

3. Blend ingredients on low, then at medium speed for 1 minute, scraping down sides of bowl with spatula as necessary. Place dough in prepared pan. Smooth top of dough with wet spatula. Cover and let rise in warm place (75–80°F) for 30–40 minutes, until dough is level with top of pan.

4. Bake at 375°F for 50–55 minutes (do not underbake). Cover with foil after 10 minutes to prevent overbrowning. Tap loaf with fingernail. A crisp, hard sound indicates a properly baked loaf. Turn loaf out onto wire rack and cool thoroughly before slicing with an electric or serrated knife.

Note: Bread will be heavier and denser without eggs.

Nutrition Information (per serving)
Calories 195 • Fat 8g • Protein 6g • Carbohydrates 28g • Cholesterol 33mg • Sodium 200mg • Fiber 1g

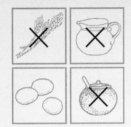

OLD-FASHIONED POTATO BREAD

Makes a 1-pound loaf (Serves 12)

So many of my customers asked me for a potato bread recipe that I finally developed this one for them.

2 teaspoons active dry yeast

2 tablespoons granulated sugar or fructose powder, divided

¾ cup warm water or potato water (110°F)

2 cups Flour Blend (page 276)

2 teaspoons xanthan gum

¾ teaspoon salt

⅓ cup dry milk powder or nondairy milk powder

¼ teaspoon soy lecithin (optional)

2 large eggs

½ cup mashed potatoes

¼ cup (½ stick) butter or spread, melted

1 teaspoon vinegar

1. All ingredients except water should be room temperature. Combine yeast, 2 teaspoons of the sugar or fructose powder, and warm water and set aside to let yeast foam, about 5 minutes.
2. In large mixer bowl using regular beaters (not dough hooks), combine flours, xanthan gum, salt, remaining sugar or fructose powder, dry milk, and soy lecithin (if using). Add eggs, mashed potatoes, melted butter, vinegar, and yeast-water mixture.
3. With mixer on low speed, beat ingredients together until blended. Beat on medium speed for 1 minute.
4. For smaller loaves, generously grease three 5x3-inch nonstick loaf pans. Divide dough among prepared pans and let rise in warm place (75–80°F) for 25–30 minutes, until dough is level with top of pan (no higher). For one large loaf, use generously greased 8x4-inch nonstick loaf pan. Let rise in warm place (75–80°F) for 45–60 minutes, until dough is level with top of pan (no higher).
5. Preheat oven to 375°F. Bake small loaves for 25–30 minutes, large loaf for 45–50 minutes, or until nicely browned.

Nutrition Information (per serving)
Calories 175 • Fat 6g • Protein 6g • Carbohydrates 29g • Cholesterol 41mg • Sodium 217mg • Fiber 0.5g

1. Have all ingredients, except water, at room temperature (about 80°F). Heat water to 110°F.
2. Once dough begins to rise in pan, don't disturb the delicate structure by shaking, dropping, or jarring pan. Don't slam oven door.
3. Rising times vary by altitude—lower altitudes may take up to 30 minutes longer.
4. Humidity, temperature, and brand of flour may affect the amount of liquid required.
5. Dough should rise to just level with top of pan before baking. If it rises much higher, it may collapse while baking.
6. Dough is proper consistency when it falls nicely off beaters in "graceful globs." If you have to pry dough off beaters, it's too dry. Add more water, 2 tablespoons at a time.

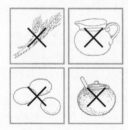

PUMPERNICKEL BREAD

This bread is great for sandwiches such as a Reuben, which is grilled in a hot skillet to a delectable crispness.

	MAKES 1 POUND	MAKES 1½ TO 2 POUNDS
	Serves 12	*Serves 18*
Active dry yeast	2¼ teaspoons	2¼ teaspoons
Milk (cow, rice, or soy) (110°F)	1 cup	1½ cups
Brown sugar or maple sugar	1 tablespoon	1½ tablespoons
Flour Blend (page 276)	2½ cups	3 cups + 1 tablespoon
Xanthan gum	1½ teaspoons	2 teaspoons

	MAKES 1 POUND	MAKES 1½ TO 2 POUNDS
Salt	1 teaspoon	1½ teaspoons
Egg replacer powder	1 teaspoon	1½ teaspoons
Caraway seeds	1 tablespoon	1½ teaspoons
Unsweetened cocoa powder	1 tablespoon	1½ tablespoons
Instant coffee powder	1 teaspoon	1½ teaspoons
Onion powder	½ teaspoon	¾ teaspoon
Eggs or silken tofu	2 large eggs, or ½ cup soft silken tofu	3 large eggs, or ¾ cup soft silken tofu
Butter (melted) or canola oil	3 tablespoons	¼ cup
Molasses or maple syrup	2 tablespoons	3 tablespoons
Vinegar	1 teaspoon	1½ teaspoons
Pans	Three 5x3-inch loaf pans, or one 9x5-inch loaf pan	Five 5x3-inch loaf pans, or two 8x4-inch loaf pans

HAND:

1. Mix yeast, milk, and sugar in bowl and set aside to let yeast foam, about 5 minutes.
2. Combine remaining dry ingredients in large mixer bowl; blend on low speed. Add eggs, butter, molasses, vinegar, and yeast mixture to dry ingredients. Beat on high for 1 minute.
3. Generously grease loaf pans. Divide dough among prepared pans and let rise in warm place (75–80°F) until dough is level with top of pan.
4. Preheat oven to 350°F. Bake small loaves for 25–30 minutes, large loaves for 40–50 minutes. Cover with foil after 10 minutes to prevent overbrowning. Tap loaf with fingernail. A crisp, hard sound indicates a properly baked loaf.

MACHINE:

Spray pan with cooking spray. Add room temperature ingredients in order listed by man-ufacturer. Set controls and bake.

Nutrition Information (per 1-inch-slice serving)
Calories 240 • Fat 6g • Protein 4g • Carbohydrates 47g • Cholesterol 33mg • Sodium 200mg • Fiber 1g

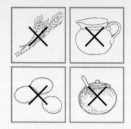

SANDWICH BREAD

This bread when made in the dairy-free, egg-free version will remind you of heavy European breads.

	MAKES 1 POUND	MAKES 2 POUNDS
	Serves 12	*Serves 18*
Active dry yeast	2¼ teaspoons	2¼ teaspoons
Brown sugar or fructose powder	1 tablespoon	2 tablespoons
Milk (cow, rice, or soy) (110°F)	1 cup	1½ cups
Flour Blend (page 276)	2½ cups	3 cups + 1 tablespoon
Xanthan gum	1½ teaspoons	2 teaspoons
Salt	1 teaspoon	1½ teaspoons
Egg replacer powder	1 teaspoon	1½ teaspoons
Eggs or silken tofu	2 large eggs, or ½ cup soft silken tofu	3 large eggs, or ¾ cup soft silken tofu
Butter (melted) or canola oil	3 tablespoons	¼ cup
Vinegar	1 teaspoon	2 teaspoons
Pans	Three 5x3-inch loaf pans, or one 9x5-inch loaf pan	Five 5x3-inch loaf pans, or two 8x4-inch loaf pans

HAND:

1. Mix yeast, sugar, and milk in bowl and set aside to let yeast foam, about 5 minutes.
2. In large mixer bowl using regular beaters, combine flour, xanthan gum, salt, and egg replacer. Add eggs, butter, vinegar, and yeast mixture.
3. Mix ingredients together on low speed, then beat on high 1 minute, scraping sides of bowl with spatula.
4. Generously grease loaf pans. Divide dough among prepared pans and let rise in warm place (75–80°F) until dough is level with top of pan.

5. Preheat oven to 350°F. Bake small loaves for 25–30 minutes, large loaves for 40–50 minutes, or until tops are nicely browned. Let cool for 5 minutes in pan. Remove from pan; cool on wire rack.

MACHINE:

Spray pan with cooking spray. Add room temperature ingredients in order listed by manufacturer. Set controls and bake.

Nutrition Information (per serving)

Calories 225 • Fat 5g • Protein 4g • Carbohydrates 44g • Cholesterol 41mg* • Sodium 227mg • Fiber 1g

*Eggs and butter add additional 56mg cholesterol per serving.

GENERAL GUIDELINES FOR MAKING BREAD WITH A BREAD MACHINE

1. Have all ingredients, including water, at room temperature (about 80°F).
2. Follow instructions for *your* bread machine. With some, add dry ingredients first, then liquid. In others, the liquid ingredients come first. Whisk dry ingredients together *thoroughly* before adding to bread machine to assure thorough blending. Whisk liquid ingredients together *thoroughly,* especially the eggs, before adding to bread machine. Some people also mix *all* ingredients together thoroughly before adding to machine.
3. Be careful not to dislodge kneading blade when scraping sides of pan.
4. With programmable machines, some experimentation may be required to achieve the right settings. My Welbilt (on light setting) warms ingredients for 20 minutes, mixes 10 minutes, rests 5 minutes, kneads 15 minutes, rises 25 minutes, punches down then rises again 54 minutes. It bakes for 40 minutes. Total time is 2 hours, 50 minutes. If you program your machine for one rise, eliminate the second rising of 54 minutes.
5. If the bread falls, there was probably too much liquid. Next time, add all but 2 tablespoons of the water and watch the dough as it kneads. If it looks dry, add water 1 tablespoon at a time. When dough is right consistency, it should swirl about in machine with a visible raised pattern on top.
6. Place the bread machine in a spot that is neither too hot nor too cold (75–80°F) for best results.
7. To assure easy removal of baked bread, grease and flour pan.

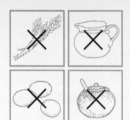

FOCACCIA

Serves 10

This is a great bread because it is a success—no matter how it turns out.

BREAD

¾ cup warm water (110°F)

1 teaspoon sugar or honey

2 large eggs, or ½ cup soft silken tofu

2 tablespoons olive oil

½ teaspoon vinegar

1½ teaspoons active dry yeast

1½ cups Flour Blend (page 276)

1 teaspoon unflavored gelatin powder

2 teaspoons xanthan gum

1 teaspoon dried rosemary leaves

½ teaspoon onion powder

¾ teaspoon salt

TOPPING

1¼ teaspoons Italian seasoning

¼ teaspoon salt

1 tablespoon olive oil

1 tablespoon grated Parmesan cheese
   (cow, rice, or soy), for garnish

BREAD:

1. In medium mixer bowl using regular beaters, combine warm water, sugar, eggs, oil, and vinegar until smooth. Add yeast, flours, gelatin, xanthan gum, rosemary, onion powder, and salt. Beat for 2 minutes. Dough will be soft and sticky.

2. Grease 11x7-inch nonstick baking pan. Transfer dough to prepared pan. Cover with foil and let rise in warm place for 30 minutes, or until dough is level with top of pan.

TOPPING:

Preheat oven to 400°F. Sprinkle focaccia with Italian seasoning, salt, and oil (or to taste). Bake for 20–25 minutes, until golden brown. Sprinkle Parmesan cheese on top.

Nutrition Information (per serving)

Calories 150 • Fat 6g • Protein 5g • Carbohydrates 23g • Cholesterol 36mg • Sodium 228mg •
   Fiber 0.5g

Topping Variations

Herb Topping: Combine ½ teaspoon *each* dried rosemary, sage, and thyme; ¼ teaspoon black pepper; and 2 tablespoons grated Parmesan cheese (cow, rice, or soy).

Calories 5 • Fat 5g • Protein 5g • Carbohydrates <1g • Cholesterol 1mg • Sodium 19mg • Fiber 0g

Sun-dried Tomato & Olive Topping: Sauté ¼ cup minced sun-dried tomatoes, ¼ cup sliced black olives, and ¼ cup chopped onion in 1 teaspoon olive oil.

Calories 100 • Fat 9g • Protein 3g • Carbohydrates 3g • Cholesterol 5mg • Sodium 480mg • Fiber 0.5g

Pesto Topping: Puree in food processor just until smooth, leaving bit of texture: 1 cup fresh basil leaves, 1 garlic clove, ½ cup pine nuts. With motor running, slowly add ¼ cup olive oil through feed tube. Add ¼ cup grated Parmesan cheese (cow, rice, or soy) and dash of black pepper.

Calories 25 • Fat 4g • Protein 0.5g • Carbohydrates 3g • Cholesterol 0mg • Sodium 1mg • Fiber 0.5g

Caramelized Onion Topping: Sprinkle focaccia dough with 1 to 2 teaspoons dried oregano, thyme, or herb of choice. Then top with 2 cups of chopped, sautéed onions that have been tossed with 1 tablespoon olive oil. Bake as directed. Serves 10.

Calories 25 • Fat 4g • Protein 1g • Carbohydrates 3g • Cholesterol 0mg • Sodium 1mg • Fiber 0.5g

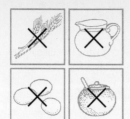

HAMBURGER BUNS

Makes 8 buns

Store these in the freezer in separate plastic bags. That way, you can take out one at a time when the urge to have a hamburger strikes. The buns will be heavier if made without eggs.

1½ teaspoons active dry yeast
1 teaspoon granulated sugar or
  fructose powder
1½ cups Flour Blend (page 276)
1½ teaspoons xanthan gum
1 teaspoon unflavored gelatin powder
1 tablespoon instant minced onion

¾ teaspoon salt
¼ teaspoon soy lecithin granules
¾ cup warm water (110°F)
2 tablespoons canola oil
2 large eggs, or ½ cup soft silken tofu
½ teaspoon vinegar

1. Combine dry ingredients in medium mixer bowl. Add warm water, oil, eggs, and vinegar and beat with electric mixer (using regular beaters, not dough hooks) for 1 minute. Dough will be soft and sticky. (Or mix in bread machine on dough setting.)
2. Grease 8 English muffin rings or aluminum foil rings (see below) and grease baking sheet. Transfer dough to prepared pans on sheet. Cover with aluminum foil and let rise in warm place for 30 minutes, or until desired height.
3. Preheat oven to 400°F. Bake for 15–20 minutes, until tops are golden brown. Cool for 5 minutes. Remove buns from rings. For crispy texture, lightly toast cut side of bun before serving.

Nutrition Information (per serving)
Calories 175 • Fat 6g • Protein 6g • Carbohydrates 28g • Cholesterol 45mg • Sodium 218mg • Fiber 0.5g

Variation

For an herb-flavored bun, add 1 teaspoon rosemary leaves (crushed) and ½ teaspoon Italian seasoning to dough.

Aluminum Foil Rings: Fold 12-inch strip of regular-size aluminum foil lengthwise into 1-inch-wide strip. Secure ends together with masking tape to form ring.

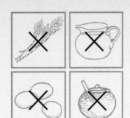

HERBED FLATBREAD

Serves 12

This easy, flavorful bread is meant to be fairly thin. You can either cut it or just tear off a piece.

BREAD

1 tablespoon dry yeast

1 cup + 2 tablespoons Flour Blend
  (page 276)

2 tablespoons dry milk powder
  or nondairy milk powder

2 teaspoons xanthan gum

½ teaspoon salt

½ teaspoon *each* caraway seeds, fennel
  seeds, dried dill weed, ground
  cumin, and dry mustard

1 teaspoon instant minced onion

½ teaspoon sugar or honey

⅔ cup warm water (110°F)

1 teaspoon olive oil

1 teaspoon vinegar

Rice flour

TOPPING

1 tablespoon olive oil

½ teaspoon coarse salt

1. In medium mixer bowl using regular beaters (not dough hooks), blend yeast, flours, milk powder, xanthan gum, salt, seeds, onion, and sugar on low speed. Add warm water, olive oil, and vinegar. Beat on high speed for 1 minute. (If the mixer bounces around the bowl, dough is too dry. Add water if necessary, 1 tablespoon at a time, until dough does not resist beaters.) Dough should resemble soft bread dough.

2. Preheat oven to 400°F. Coat 15x10-inch nonstick jelly-roll pan with cooking spray. Place dough in prepared pan. Liberally sprinkle rice flour on dough, then press dough into pan with hands, continuing to sprinkle dough with rice flour to prevent sticking to hands. Dough should extend up to within 1 inch of pan edge, but should not touch edge of pan.

3. Brush with olive oil. Sprinkle with coarse salt. Bake for 15–20 minutes, or golden brown and edges are turned up. Remove from oven. Cut or tear into pieces.

Note: You can make your own dry mustard by grinding mustard seeds in a small coffee grinder.

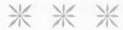

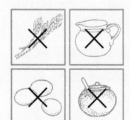

ITALIAN BREAD STICKS

Serves 10

Breadsticks are one of the easiest ways to serve bread at any meal. For an attractive presentation, stand the sticks on end in a decorative pitcher or container.

1 tablespoon active dry yeast	1 tablespoon dry milk powder
⅔ cup warm 2% milk (cow, rice, or soy) (110°F)	or nondairy powder
½ teaspoon sugar or honey	½ teaspoon salt
½ cup brown rice flour or sorghum flour	1 teaspoon onion powder
½ cup tapioca flour	1 teaspoon unflavored gelatin powder
2 teaspoons xanthan gum	1 tablespoon olive oil
½ cup grated Parmesan cheese (cow, rice, or soy)	1 teaspoon vinegar
	1 large egg white, beaten to foam, or cooking spray
	1 teaspoon Italian seasoning

1. Mix yeast, milk, and sugar in small bowl and set aside to let yeast foam, about 5 minutes.
2. Preheat oven to 400°F for 5 minutes, then turn off.
3. In medium-size mixer bowl, blend yeast-milk mixture, flours, xanthan gum, Parmesan cheese, dry milk powder, salt, onion powder, gelatin, oil, and vinegar on low speed of electric mixer. Beat on high for 1 minute. Dough will be soft and sticky.

4. Place dough in large, heavy-duty plastic freezer bag with ½-inch opening cut diagonally on one corner. (This makes a 1-inch circle.) Grease large nonstick baking sheet. Squeeze dough out of plastic bag onto sheet in 10 strips, each 1 inch wide by 6 inches long. For best results, hold bag of dough upright as you squeeze, rather than at an angle. Also, hold bag with corners perpendicular, rather than horizontal, to baking sheet for more authentic-looking bread stick. Brush with beaten egg white or spray with cooking spray for crispier, shinier bread stick. Sprinkle with Italian seasoning.

5. Let rise in warmed oven for 20–30 minutes. Then, while bread sticks remain in oven, turn oven to 400°F and bake about 15–20 minutes, until golden brown. Rotate baking sheet halfway through baking to assure even browning. Cool on wire rack.

Nutrition Information (per bread stick)
Calories 85 • Fat 3g • Protein 3g • Carbohydrates 13g • Cholesterol 3mg • Sodium 192mg • Fiber 1g

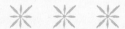

 QUICK BREADS

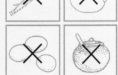

BACON-ONION MUFFINS

Makes 12 muffins

These tasty muffins are best eaten right after they come out of the oven.

3 cups Flour Blend (page 276)	1½ teaspoons xanthan gum
1 tablespoon baking powder	1 teaspoon salt
1 tablespoon sugar or honey	1 teaspoon dried thyme leaves
1½ teaspoons unflavored gelatin powder	1 cup 2% milk (cow, rice, or soy)

¼ cup canola oil

3 large eggs, or ¾ cup soft silken tofu

¼ cup finely chopped cooked bacon

1 tablespoon dried minced onion

1. Preheat oven to 400°F. Grease standard 12-cup muffin pan.
2. Combine all dry ingredients in medium mixer bowl. Add milk, oil, and eggs and beat with electric mixer until smooth. Stir in bacon and onion.
3. Divide evenly in prepared muffin pan, filling each indentation to just below top.
4. Bake for 20–25 minutes, or until tops are golden brown and crusty. Serve immediately.

Nutrition Information (per muffin)

Calories 295 • Fat 8g • Protein 5g • Carbohydrates 54g • Cholesterol 48mg • Sodium 396mg • Fiber 0.5g

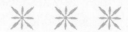

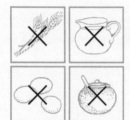

QUICK-BREAD BREAD STICKS

Makes 10 bread sticks

These bread sticks are best when eaten right after they come out of the oven.

BREAD STICKS

¾ cup brown rice flour or garbanzo/ fava bean flour

¼ cup sweet rice flour

2 tablespoons tapioca flour

1 teaspoon xanthan gum

1 teaspoon sugar or honey

1½ teaspoons baking powder

½ teaspoon salt

½ teaspoon onion powder

¼ teaspoon potato flour (not potato starch)

¼ teaspoon Italian seasoning

¾ cup 2% milk (cow, rice, or soy)

Cooking spray
¼ **teaspoon salt**
1 **teaspoon Italian seasoning**
2 **teaspoons sesame seeds (optional)**

1. Preheat oven to 425°F. Grease large nonstick baking sheet and set aside.
2. Combine all bread stick ingredients in food processor. Blend thoroughly. Dough will be soft.
3. Place dough in large, heavy-duty plastic freezer bag that has ½-inch opening cut diagonally on one corner. (This makes a 1-inch diameter opening.) Squeeze dough out of plastic bag onto prepared baking sheet in 10 strips, each 1 inch wide by 6 inches long. Hold the bag of dough upright as you squeeze, rather than at an angle. Also, hold bag with seam on top, rather than at side.
4. Spray bread sticks with cooking spray. Sprinkle with salt, Italian seasoning, and sesame seeds (if using).
5. Bake for 15–20 minutes, until browned. Switch position of baking sheet halfway through baking for even browning. Cool on wire rack. Store bread sticks in an airtight container to maintain softness.

Nutrition Information (per bread stick)
Calories 90 • Fat 1g • Protein 2g • Carbohydrates 18g • Cholesterol 2mg • Sodium 225mg • Fiber 0.5g

Note: If using electric mixer instead of food processor, add 2 tablespoons of water so batter is consistency of soft cookie dough.

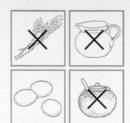

CORN BREAD

Serves 12

Some corn bread experts insist on baking corn bread in a preheated 9-inch cast-iron skillet. That method works fine with this recipe, producing a slightly crispy crust.

1¼ cups cornmeal

1 cup Flour Blend (page 276)

⅓ cup granulated sugar or fructose powder

2 teaspoons baking powder

1½ teaspoons xanthan gum

1 teaspoon salt

2 large eggs*

1 cup 2% milk (cow, rice, or soy)

⅓ cup canola oil

1. Preheat oven to 375°F. Grease 8-inch square nonstick baking pan or 9-inch cast-iron skillet and set aside.
2. In medium mixer bowl, combine cornmeal, flours, sugar or fructose powder, baking powder, xanthan gum, and salt. Make well in center.
3. In another bowl, beat eggs, milk, and oil until well blended. Add egg mixture all at once to dry mixture, stirring just until moistened. Pour mixture into prepared pan.
4. Bake for 20–25 minutes, until top is firm and edges are lightly browned. Serve warm.

Nutrition Information (per serving)

Calories 215 • Fat 8g • Protein 4g • Carbohydrates 35g • Cholesterol 32mg • Sodium 258mg • Fiber 1g

Variation

Corn Bread with Green Chiles: Gently stir in 2 tablespoons chopped fresh cilantro and 1 can (4 ounces) diced green chiles after ingredients are mixed together. If you are not accustomed to eating green chiles, you might reduce the amount to 2 tablespoons the first time you make this corn bread.

Calories 220 • Fat 8g • Protein 4g • Carbohydrates 35g • Cholesterol 32mg • Sodium 258mg • Fiber 1.5g

*Corn Bread Without Eggs: Omit egg, and add 2 teaspoons egg replacer powder and increase milk to 1 cup. Bake for 20–25 minutes, until top is firm and lightly browned.

Calories 150 • Fat 4g • Protein 4g • Carbohydrates 25g • Cholesterol 32mg • Sodium 258mg • Fiber 1g

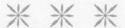

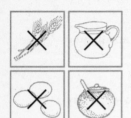

IRISH GRIDDLE CAKES

Serves 6

This is a great way to use up leftover mashed potatoes, and it provides a crispy, chewy bread in relatively little time.

1 cup mashed potatoes	½ teaspoon baking powder
¾ cup Flour Blend (page 276)	1 tablespoon canola oil
½ teaspoon xanthan gum	1 tablespoon 2% milk (cow, rice,
½ teaspoon salt	or soy)
½ teaspoon crushed dried rosemary	Rice flour
leaves	1 tablespoon canola oil, for frying
½ teaspoon onion powder	

1. Combine all ingredients except oil for frying in food processor until thoroughly mixed. Roll out between sheets of waxed paper into ¼-inch-thick circle. Dust with additional rice flour to prevent sticking.
2. With sharp knife, cut circle in half, then cut each half into 3 wedges.
3. Heat griddle or cast-iron skillet until medium-hot. Add oil and fry cakes for 5–7 minutes on each side, until golden brown, turning once. Serve hot.

Nutrition Information (per serving)
Calories 180 • Fat 6g • Protein 2g • Carbohydrates 32g • Cholesterol 1mg • Sodium 301mg • Fiber 0.5g

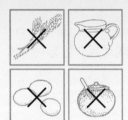

IRISH SODA BREAD

Serves 10

Serve this bread with your favorite Irish meal. It is also great just on its own. The dried tart cherries are not traditional but provide a contemporary touch. You can omit them, if you wish.

2 cups Flour Blend (page 276)

2 teaspoons granulated sugar or fructose powder

1 teaspoon xanthan gum

¾ teaspoon salt

½ teaspoon unflavored gelatin powder

½ teaspoon baking powder

½ teaspoon baking soda

1 large egg, or ¼ cup soft silken tofu

1 cup buttermilk, or 2 tablespoons vinegar or lemon juice and enough nondairy milk to equal 1 cup

2 tablespoons canola oil

1 tablespoon caraway seeds

1. Preheat oven to 350°F. Grease two 5x3-inch nonstick loaf pans or one 8-inch square nonstick baking pan.
2. Combine dry ingredients in large mixer bowl and mix well. With electric mixer on low, add egg, buttermilk, oil, and caraway seeds. Blend on medium speed for 2 minutes.
3. Spoon into prepared pan(s), smoothing tops with wet spatula if necessary. Bake small pans for 45–50 minutes, large pan for 50–55 minutes, until top is deeply browned and loaf sounds hollow when tapped. Cool on wire rack. Slice with serrated knife or electric knife when bread reaches room temperature.

Nutrition Information (per serving)
Calories 215 • Fat 5g • Protein 3g • Carbohydrates 44g • Cholesterol 2mg • Sodium 245mg • Fiber 0.5g

Variation

Irish Soda Bread with Dried Cherries: Gently stir in ½ cup chopped dried cherries after the ingredients are mixed.

Calories 225 • Fat 5g • Protein 4g • Carbohydrates 45g • Cholesterol 2mg • Sodium 245mg • Fiber 1g

QUICK-BREAD FOCACCIA

Serves 10

This recipe often becomes a big favorite for those on yeast-free diets. The focaccia can be dipped in herbed olive oil, split horizontally for sandwiches, or split and toasted much like a bagel.

BREAD

2 cups Flour Blend (page 276)

2 teaspoons sugar or honey

2 teaspoons xanthan gum

¾ teaspoon salt

½ teaspoon unflavored gelatin powder

1 teaspoon baking powder

1¼ teaspoons baking soda

¾ teaspoon onion powder

1 teaspoon crushed dried rosemary

¼ teaspoon potato flour (not potato starch)

2 large eggs, or ½ cup soft silken tofu

1 cup 2% milk (cow, rice, or soy)

2 tablespoons olive oil

TOPPING

1 tablespoon olive oil

1½ teaspoons Italian seasoning

½ teaspoon salt

2 tablespoons grated Parmesan cheese (cow, rice, or soy—optional)

1. Preheat oven to 375°F. Grease one 11x7-inch nonstick baking pan, or two 8-inch round nonstick baking pans, or one 13x9-inch nonstick baking pan. (Use 11x7-inch pan or 8-inch pans for thicker bread to slice horizontally for sandwiches. Use 13x9-inch pan for thinner bread to use as pizza crust.)

2. Combine dry ingredients in large mixer bowl. With electric mixer on low, add eggs, milk, and oil and blend on medium speed for 1 minute. Dough will be soft and sticky. Spread batter in prepared pan(s) with wet spatula. Sprinkle with olive oil, Italian seasoning, and salt.

3. Bake for 20–25 minutes, until top is well browned. Dust with Parmesan cheese (if using).

Serving Suggestions: Cut into 3-inch squares or slice entire round loaf horizontally, then place sandwich fillings on bottom half and replace top half. Slice into wedges and serve. Or use the focaccia as yeast-free pizza crust with your favorite toppings. See Focaccia Toppings on pages 23–24.

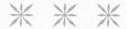

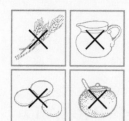

QUICK-BREAD HAMBURGER BUNS

Makes 8 buns

Bake a batch, freeze them individually in plastic bags, and defrost them when the hamburgers come off the grill.

2 cups Flour Blend (page 276)
1 tablespoon dried minced onion
2 teaspoons sugar or honey
2 teaspoons xanthan gum
1¼ teaspoons baking soda
1 teaspoon baking powder
¾ teaspoon salt
½ teaspoon unflavored gelatin powder

¼ teaspoon soy lecithin granules
1 teaspoon butter-flavored extract (optional)
2 large eggs, or ½ cup soft silken tofu
1 cup 2% milk (cow, rice, or soy)
2 tablespoons canola oil
2 teaspoons sesame seeds (optional)

1. Preheat oven to 375°F. Spray eight 4-inch English muffin or aluminum foil rings on nonstick baking pan with cooking spray. (See page 25 for making aluminum foil rings.)

2. Combine dry ingredients in large mixer bowl. With electric mixer on low, add eggs, milk, and oil and blend on medium speed for 2 minutes. Dough will be soft and sticky.

3. Spoon into 8 prepared rings; smooth tops with wet spatula. Sprinkle with sesame seeds (if using). Bake for 15–20 minutes, until tops are lightly browned. (For extra-large or extra-small buns, make your own aluminum foil rings in desired size.)

Nutrition Information (per bun)

Calories 230 • Fat 7g • Protein 7g • Carbohydrates 39g • Cholesterol 27mg • Sodium 470mg • Fiber 0g

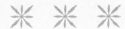

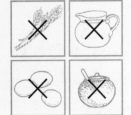

HEARTY SANDWICH BREAD

Serves 12

This bread produces a better crust and more palatable texture when baked in two 5x3-inch pans rather than one 9x5-inch pan.

1¾ cups Flour Blend (page 276)

⅓ cup almond meal/flour*

⅓ cup rice bran

2 tablespoons light brown sugar or maple sugar

1 teaspoon salt

2 teaspoons baking powder

¼ teaspoon potato flour (not potato starch)

2 large eggs, or ½ cup soft silken tofu

¾ cup 2% milk (cow, rice, or soy)

¼ cup canola oil

*Purchase in natural food stores, or grind almonds in electric coffee grinder until fine—but stop before they turn into butter.

1. Preheat oven to 350°F. Grease one 9x5-inch nonstick loaf pan or two 5x3-inch non-stick baking pans.

2. Combine dry ingredients in large mixer bowl. Add remaining ingredients and mix with electric mixer on low until well blended.

3. Transfer batter to prepared pan(s) and smooth tops with wet spatula. Bake small loaves for 45–50 minutes, large loaf for 50–55 minutes, or until crust sounds hard when tapped. Don't underbake.

4. Cool in pan for 5 minutes, then cool completely on wire rack before slicing with electric or serrated knife.

Nutrition Information (per serving)
Calories 210 • Fat 7g • Protein 4g • Carbohydrates 35g • Cholesterol 32mg • Sodium 255mg • Fiber 1g

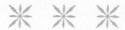

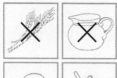

QUICK-BREAD PIZZA CRUST

Serves 6

This won't have the chewy crust found in yeasted pizza crusts, but it is still a treat to have pizza when you can't eat yeast. You can use pizza sauce of your choice or see page 161 for a flavorful recipe.

½ cup cornstarch or potato starch
½ cup tapioca flour
1 teaspoon sugar or honey
1 teaspoon xanthan gum
½ teaspoon salt
¼ teaspoon potato flour (not potato starch)
1 teaspoon baking powder
½ teaspoon onion powder

½ teaspoon dried rosemary leaves
½ teaspoon Italian seasoning
2 tablespoons butter or margarine
1 large egg, or 1 tablespoon egg replacer powder mixed in 3 tablespoons water
¼ cup 2% milk (cow, rice, or soy)
Rice flour

1. Preheat oven to 400°F. Grease 12-inch nonstick pizza pan (for a thin, crispy crust) or 11x7-inch nonstick baking pan or 10-inch cast-iron skillet (for a deep-dish crust).
2. In food processor, combine all ingredients except egg, milk, and rice flour. Blend until mixture resembles fine bread crumbs. Add egg and milk and process until dough forms ball. Dough will be stiff, but sticky.
3. Place dough on prepared pan and sprinkle with rice flour. Pat dough to ¼-inch thickness with hands—just up to edges of pan, sprinkling more rice flour as needed to prevent sticking. Make dough slightly higher around outer edge to contain toppings. Bake for 10–15 minutes. Remove from oven and top with toppings. Bake for another 10–15 minutes, or until browned to taste.

Nutrition Information (per serving)
Calories 130 • Fat 6g • Protein 2g • Carbohydrates 20g • Cholesterol 33mg • Sodium 230mg • Fiber 0.5g

Note: For a smoother crust, replace 2 tablespoons of cornstarch with dry milk powder (dairy or nondairy).

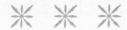

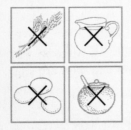

QUICK-BREAD SANDWICH BREAD

Serves 12

The reason this bread is baked in smaller pans is that it produces a better crust and a better texture than if it is baked in a larger pan.

2¼ cups Flour Blend (page 276)
3 tablespoons sugar or honey
2 teaspoons xanthan gum

2 teaspoons baking powder
1 teaspoon salt
½ teaspoon unflavored gelatin powder

¼ teaspoon potato flour (not potato starch)	1 cup 2% milk (cow, rice, or soy)
2 large eggs, or ½ cup silken tofu	¼ cup (½ stick) butter (melted) or canola oil

1. Preheat oven to 375°F. Grease two 5x3-inch nonstick loaf pans or one 9x5-inch non-stick loaf pan.
2. Combine dry ingredients in large mixer bowl. With electric mixer on low, add remaining ingredients and mix until smooth.
3. Spoon into prepared pan(s) and smooth top with wet spatula if necessary. Bake small pans for 45–50 minutes, large pan for 50–55 minutes, until top is deeply browned and loaf sounds crisp when tapped. Don't underbake. Cool completely on wire rack before slicing with serrated or electric knife.

Nutrition Information (per serving)
Calories 250 • Fat 10g • Protein 3g • Carbohydrates 41g • Cholesterol 40mg • Sodium 286mg • Fiber 0.5g

Quick-Bread Dill-Onion Bread: Add 1 teaspoon dill weed, 1½ tablespoons dill seed, and 1 tablespoon dried minced onion.

Other Variations

Tailor this basic bread to suit your individual tastes and dietary needs. For more fiber, add sesame seeds, rice bran, or rice polish (available from Ener-G Foods—see References) and subtract equivalent amount of rice or bean flour. For additional flavor, add 1 tablespoon minced onion and butter-flavored extract. For herb bread, add 1–2 teaspoons (or more, to taste) of your favorite dried herbs or spices.

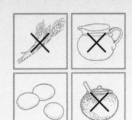

SPOON BREAD

Serves 8

This is an easy bread that turns out well because it's supposed to be soft and spooned rather than cut.

2 large eggs

1 cup plain yogurt, or ¾ cup 2% milk
  (cow, rice, or soy)

½ cup finely chopped onion

2 tablespoons canola oil

1 can (4 ounces) diced green chiles
  (optional)

¾ cup yellow cornmeal

1 teaspoon baking powder

1 teaspoon garlic salt

1 cup corn kernels

1 cup shredded low-fat cheddar cheese
  (cow or soy)

1. Preheat oven to 350°F. Grease 9-inch cast-iron skillet or 9-inch round or square non-stick baking pan.
2. Beat eggs with wire whisk in large bowl. Add yogurt, onion, oil, and chiles (if using) and mix well.
3. In another bowl, combine cornmeal, baking powder, and garlic salt. Add to egg mixture. Stir in corn and ½ cup of cheddar cheese. (If using soy cheddar cheese, add all cheese to batter, since it might not melt on top.) Batter will be soft.
4. Pour batter into prepared pans. Sprinkle remaining ½ cup cheese (if using cow's-milk cheese) over top. Bake for 40–50 minutes, until top is golden brown. Spoon out of pan.

Nutrition Information (per serving)

Calories 170 • Fat 6g • Protein 8g • Carbohydrates 18g • Cholesterol 50mg • Sodium 208mg •
  Fiber 2g

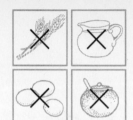

ZUCCHINI BREAD

Serves 12

This bread is a great way to use up all those zucchini in your garden.

¼ cup canola oil
⅔ cup packed light brown sugar or
    maple sugar*
2 large eggs, or ½ cup soft silken tofu
1 teaspoon vanilla extract
½ cup drained applesauce
1¾ cups Flour Blend (page 276)
2 teaspoons baking powder

1 teaspoon xanthan gum
½ teaspoon salt
1½ teaspoons ground cinnamon
1½ cups grated zucchini (3 small
    zucchini)
½ cup chopped pecans (optional)
¼ cup dark raisins (optional)

1. Preheat oven to 350°F. Grease one 9x5-inch nonstick loaf pan or three 5x3-inch nonstick loaf pans.
2. In large bowl, combine oil and sugar with electric mixer. Add eggs, vanilla, and applesauce and beat until very smooth. Add flours, baking powder, xanthan gum, salt, and cinnamon. Mix on medium speed until thoroughly combined. Quickly (but gently) stir in zucchini (and nuts and raisins, if using). Batter will be thick. Turn batter into prepared pan(s).
3. Bake 9x5-inch loaf for 1 hour, 5x3-inch pans for 45 minutes. Cool on wire rack before cutting.

Nutrition Information (per serving)
Calories 240 • Fat 7g • Protein 3g • Carbohydrates 44g • Cholesterol 30mg • Sodium 163mg •
    Fiber 1g

Note: If raisins and nuts are omitted, use two instead of three 5x3-inch pans because volume of bread is considerably reduced.

*Sugar Alternative: Use ⅓ cup honey in place of ⅔ cup packed light brown sugar. Add ½ teaspoon baking soda.

BREAKFAST & BRUNCH

Breakfast can be the most frustrating meal of the day for those of us on gluten-free diets. It just isn't breakfast without bagels, muffins, waffles, or pancakes, but all of these foods contain wheat. You can enjoy gluten-free versions of your breakfast favorites—without dairy or eggs, if necessary—with the recipes in this chapter.

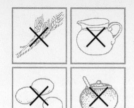

BAGELS

Makes 8 bagels

Who can resist a hot, chewy bagel—fresh from the oven?!

1 cup garbanzo/fava bean flour or
   sorghum flour
¾ cup brown rice flour
¾ cup potato starch
½ cup cornstarch
1 tablespoon active dry yeast
1 tablespoon xanthan gum
1 teaspoon salt
1 cup warm water (110°F)
2 tablespoons canola oil

2 tablespoons honey
1 large egg, lightly beaten,
   or ¼ cup Flax Mix
   (page 108)
1 teaspoon vinegar
Rice flour
1 teaspoon granulated sugar
1 egg white, beaten to a foam
   (optional)

1. Combine dry ingredients in large mixer bowl. Add liquid ingredients. Beat with electric mixer on medium for 2 minutes. Mixture will be very thick and stiff.
2. Place dough on flat, floured surface and dust dough with rice flour to make it easier to handle. Divide dough into 8 equal balls. Dust each portion with rice flour, shape each portion into ball, then flatten to 3-inch circle and punch hole in center, continuing to dust with flour, if necessary. Form into bagel shapes (turning rough edges of dough to underside) and place on large greased baking sheet.
3. Place sheet in *cold* oven. Turn to 325°F and bake for 15 minutes.
4. Meanwhile, bring 3 inches of water and sugar to boil in deep skillet. Boil bagels on each side for 30 seconds. (Leave oven on.) Using slotted spoon, return bagels to greased baking sheet. Brush with optional egg white wash to produce shinier, crispier crust.
5. Return baking sheet to oven; increase temperature to 400°F. Bake for 20–25 minutes, or until nicely browned. Remove bagels and cool on wire rack.

Nutrition Information (per bagel)
Calories 275 • Fat 6g • Protein 8g • Carbohydrates 37g • Cholesterol 23mg • Sodium 294mg •
   Fiber 2g

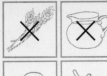

ENGLISH MUFFINS

Makes 12 muffins

These are great on their own, toasted and slathered with jam, or as the basis for Eggs Benedict.

2 tablespoons active dry yeast

2⅓ cups brown rice flour or sorghum flour

2 cups tapioca flour

⅔ cup dry milk powder or nondairy milk powder

3 teaspoons xanthan gum

1 tablespoon unflavored gelatin powder

1 teaspoon salt

1 tablespoon sugar or honey

¼ cup canola oil

4 large egg whites, or ½ cup soft silken tofu

1¼ cups warm water (110°F)

1. Have ingredients at room temperature. Combine dry ingredients in large mixer bowl. Add oil, eggs, and water (and honey, if using); beat on high for 2 minutes.

2. Arrange 12 greased muffin rings or aluminum foil rings (see page 25) on greased baking sheet. Divide dough into 12 equal balls and press into each ring. Cover and let rise in a warm place for about 50 minutes, or until dough is not quite level with top of ring.

3. Preheat oven to 350°F. Bake for 15 minutes, or until lightly browned. With spatula, turn muffins (tins and all) over and bake for another 10 minutes, or until lightly browned. Remove from baking sheet to cool. When rings are cool enough to handle, remove muffins from rings and cool on wire rack.

Nutrition Information (per muffin made with eggs)

Calories 240 • Fat 6g • Protein 6g • Carbohydrates 46g • Cholesterol 1mg • Sodium 224mg • Fiber 2g

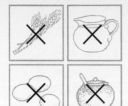

BLUEBERRY MUFFINS

Makes 12 muffins

These delightful muffins are perfect for everyday or special breakfasts or brunches. Sprinkle the muffins with Streusel Topping (see page 46).

MUFFINS

2⅓ cups Flour Blend (page 276)

½ cup granulated sugar or fructose powder

2½ teaspoons baking powder

1 teaspoon xanthan gum

1 teaspoon unflavored gelatin powder

1 teaspoon salt

1 cup 2% milk (cow, rice, or soy)

¼ cup canola oil

2 large eggs, or ½ cup soft silken tofu

1 teaspoon vanilla extract

1 tablespoon grated lemon zest

1 cup blueberries, fresh or frozen

GLAZE

2 tablespoons powdered sugar or fructose powder

2 tablespoons fresh lemon juice

1. Preheat oven to 400°F. Grease 12-cup nonstick muffin tin.
2. In large mixer bowl with electric mixer, combine dry ingredients. Add milk, oil, eggs, vanilla, and lemon zest and blend on medium until ingredients are thoroughly moistened. Gently stir in blueberries. (If the blueberries are frozen, add 5 minutes to baking time.)
3. Divide batter equally among cups in prepared muffin tin. Bake for 20–25 minutes, until tops of muffins are lightly browned. Remove from oven and cool on wire rack.
4. While muffins cool in tin, combine sugar or fructose powder and lemon juice to form glaze. Drizzle over warm muffins. Cool for 15 minutes, then remove muffins from tin. Serve immediately.

Nutrition Information (per muffin made with eggs)

Calories 270 • Fat 6g • Protein 3g • Carbohydrates 52g • Cholesterol 33mg • Sodium 274mg • Fiber 1g

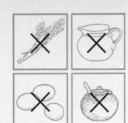

STREUSEL TOPPING FOR MUFFINS & CAKES

Makes 12 servings

Keep this on hand in your refrigerator and use it on any type of muffin or on your favorite coffee cake.

 2 tablespoons brown rice flour
 ¼ cup brown sugar or maple sugar
 ½ teaspoon ground cinnamon
 ¼ cup chopped pecans
 1 tablespoon canola oil

Combine ingredients thoroughly. Sprinkle topping evenly on muffins before baking.

Nutrition Information (per 2-tablespoon serving)
Calories 40 • Fat 2.5g • Protein <1g • Carbohydrates 4g • Cholesterol 0mg • Sodium 1mg •
  Fiber <1g

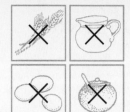

MUFFIN MIXES

Makes 4 batches (48 muffins)

These easy muffin mixes save time because you just add the liquid ingredients. They're also more economical than store-bought muffin mixes, and you have the flexibility of choosing the flours to suit your taste. For savory dinner or luncheon muffins, reduce the sugar in any of these recipes and add your favorite herbs and spices.

RICE FLOUR MUFFIN MIX

4 cups brown rice flour

2⅔ cups potato starch

2⅔ cups tapioca flour

2 cups granulated sugar or fructose
    powder

4 tablespoons baking powder

4 teaspoons xanthan gum

4 teaspoons unflavored gelatin
    powder

3½ teaspoons salt

Mix all ingredients together and store in airtight container.

BEAN SORGHUM FLOUR MUFFIN MIX

4 cups potato starch or cornstarch

3⅓ cups garbanzo/fava bean flour

2 cups granulated sugar or fructose
    powder

1 cup tapioca flour

1 cup sorghum flour

4 teaspoons unflavored gelatin powder

3½ teaspoons salt

Mix all ingredients together and store in an airtight container.

SORGHUM FLOUR MUFFIN MIX

9⅓ cups Flour Blend
    (page 276)

2 cups granulated sugar or fructose
    powder

4 tablespoons baking powder

4 teaspoons unflavored gelatin powder

4 teaspoons xanthan gum

3½ teaspoons salt

Mix all ingredients together and store in an airtight container.

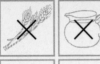

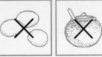

YOUR FAVORITE MUFFINS

Makes 12 muffins

2⅓ cups any Muffin Mix
¼ cup canola oil
2 large eggs, or ½ cup soft silken tofu
1 teaspoon vanilla extract
1 cup 2% milk (cow, rice, or soy)
Berries of choice, lemon zest, and/or
    poppy seeds (optional)

GLAZE (OPTIONAL)
2 tablespoons powdered sugar or
    fructose powder
2 tablespoons fresh lemon juice

1. Preheat oven to 400°F. Grease standard 12-cup nonstick muffin tin (2-inch-diameter base), or use paper liners, and set aside.
2. Put muffin mix in large mixer bowl. Add oil, eggs, vanilla, and milk and beat with electric mixer on medium speed until smooth. Gently stir in additional ingredients (blueberries, lemon zest, poppy seeds, etc.). Spoon dough into prepared muffin tin.
3. Bake for 25–35 minutes (bake 5 minutes longer if using frozen blueberries), until muffin tops are lightly browned. Remove from oven. Combine powdered sugar and lemon juice to form glaze (if using). Drizzle over warm muffins.

Nutrition Information (per muffin)
Calories 210 • Fat 7g • Protein 3g • Carbohydrates 36g • Cholesterol 32mg • Sodium 228mg •
    Fiber 1g

Variation

Lemon Poppy-Seed Muffins: Add 3 tablespoons grated lemon zest and 2 tablespoons poppy seeds.

Note: Muffins without added nuts or fruit (e.g., blueberries, cranberries, etc.) have less volume and therefore are smaller.

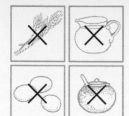

BRAN MUFFINS

Makes 12 muffins

If you prefer a hearty muffin for breakfast, but one that isn't too sweet—this muffin is for you. If you like to bake only a few muffins at a time, this batter keeps in the refrigerator for up to two days. If you omit the raisins and nuts, the muffins will be somewhat smaller.

2⅓ cups Flour Blend (page 276)
¼ cup rice bran
1½ teaspoons ground cinnamon
1¼ teaspoons xanthan gum
¾ teaspoon baking soda
¾ teaspoon salt
½ teaspoon ground ginger
½ teaspoon ground allspice
¼ teaspoon ground nutmeg
1 cup 2% milk (cow, rice, or soy)

3 tablespoons vinegar or fresh
   lemon juice
2 large eggs, or ½ cup soft silken tofu
¼ cup canola oil
½ cup molasses or maple syrup
1 teaspoon vanilla extract
⅔ cup raisins (optional)
⅓ cup chopped walnuts (optional)
1 tablespoon grated orange zest

1. Preheat oven to 375°F. Grease 12-cup standard nonstick muffin tin.
2. Combine flours with other dry ingredients in large mixer bowl. Add milk, vinegar, eggs, oil, molasses, and vanilla and use electric mixer to mix until very smooth. Gently stir in raisins and nuts (if using), and orange zest.
3. Divide batter equally among prepared muffin cups. Bake for 20–25 minutes, until tops of muffins are firm and lightly browned. Remove from oven. Cool muffins in tin for 10 minutes, then remove from tin. Serve warm.

Nutrition Information (per muffin)
Calories 290 • Fat 7g • Protein 4g • Carbohydrates 57g • Cholesterol 37mg • Sodium 237mg • Fiber 1.5g

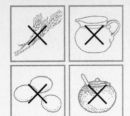

CAPPUCCINO CHOCOLATE-CHIP MUFFINS

Makes 12 muffins

These delicious muffins combine two favorite flavors—coffee and chocolate. They travel well and are sure to delight your chocoholic friends and family. For an added touch after the muffins are baked, sprinkle the tops with Dutch cocoa power or chocolate sprinkles, available from Miss Roben's (Allergy Grocer)—see Resources.

1¼ cups Flour Blend (page 276)

1 cup unsweetened cocoa powder (not Dutch process)

⅔ cup packed light brown sugar or maple sugar

1½ teaspoons xanthan gum

1 teaspoon unflavored gelatin powder

1 teaspoon instant coffee granules or espresso powder

1 teaspoon ground cinnamon

1 teaspoon salt

½ teaspoon baking soda

½ cup 2% milk (cow, rice, or soy)

½ cup warm brewed coffee (110°F)

¼ cup canola oil

2 large eggs, or ½ cup soft silken tofu

1 teaspoon vanilla extract

½ cup gluten-free, dairy-free chocolate chips

¼ cup finely chopped nuts of your choice

1. Preheat oven to 375°F. Grease 12-cup nonstick muffin tin.
2. In large bowl, combine flours, cocoa, sugar, xanthan gum, gelatin, coffee granules, cinnamon, salt, and baking soda. Add milk, coffee, oil, eggs or tofu, and vanilla and beat with electric mixer on medium speed until thoroughly blended. Gently stir in chocolate chips and nuts.
3. Divide batter equally among prepared muffin cups. Bake for 20–25 minutes, until tops of muffins are very firm. Remove from oven. Serve slightly warm so chocolate chips are still soft.

Nutrition Information (per muffin made with eggs)

Calories 240 • Fat 11g • Protein 4g • Carbohydrates 39g • Cholesterol 31mg • Sodium 251mg • Fiber 3.5g

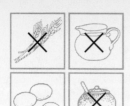

SCONES

Makes 8 scones

Scones are foolproof because any way you make them they're a success. For Scones Without Eggs, see page 53.

¼ cup (½ stick) butter or margarine

⅔ cup plain yogurt, or ½ cup 2% milk (cow, rice, or soy)

1 large egg

1¼ cups brown rice flour or sorghum flour

½ cup tapioca flour

2 tablespoons granulated sugar or fructose powder

1½ teaspoons cream of tartar

1 teaspoon xanthan gum

¾ teaspoon baking soda

½ teaspoon salt

¼ teaspoon soy lecithin (optional)

½ cup currants

1. Preheat oven to 425°F. Grease baking sheet or line with parchment paper.
2. In food processor, blend butter, yogurt, and egg until well mixed. Add flours, sugar or fructose powder, cream of tartar, xanthan gum, baking soda, salt, and lecithin (if using). Process just until mixed. Add currants and pulse a few times to incorporate. Dough will be soft.
3. Transfer dough to prepared baking sheet, patting with spatula into 8-inch circle, ¾ inch thick. Bake for 15–20 minutes, until deeply browned. For crispier, wedge-shaped pieces, cut into 8 wedges and return to oven for the final 5 minutes of baking.

Nutrition Information (per scone)
Calories 215 • Fat 7g • Protein 4g • Carbohydrates 38g • Cholesterol 38mg • Sodium 333mg • Fiber 2g

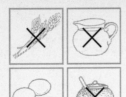

SCONES WITH HAM

Makes 8 scones

Studded with tasty morsels of ham, these hearty scones are almost a meal by themselves.

¼ cup (½ stick) butter or margarine

⅔ cup plain yogurt, or ½ cup 2% milk (cow, rice, or soy)

1 large egg

1¼ cups sorghum flour

½ cup tapioca flour

2 tablespoons granulated sugar or fructose powder

1½ teaspoons dried sage leaves

1½ teaspoons cream of tartar

1 teaspoon xanthan gum

¾ teaspoon baking soda

½ teaspoon salt

½ cup diced ham

1. Preheat oven to 425°F. Grease nonstick baking sheet or line with parchment paper.
2. In food processor, blend butter, yogurt, and egg until well mixed. Add flours, sugar, sage, cream of tartar, xanthan gum, baking soda, and salt. Process just until mixed. Remove bowl from stand and quickly stir in diced ham. Dough will be soft.
3. Transfer dough to prepared sheet, patting with spatula into 8-inch circle, ¾ inch thick. Bake for 15–20 minutes, until deeply browned. For crispier, wedge-shaped pieces, cut into 8 wedges and return to oven for the final 5 minutes of baking.

Nutrition Information (per scone)
Calories 215 • Fat 8g • Protein 5g • Carbohydrates 31g • Cholesterol 46mg • Sodium 390mg • Fiber 2g

Scones with Sun-dried Tomatoes & Olives: Omit sage and chopped ham. Add 1 teaspoon crushed rosemary leaves, ½ cup chopped sun-dried tomatoes, and ½ cup sliced black olives. Bake as directed above.

Calories 220 • Fat 8g • Protein 4g • Carbohydrates 33g • Cholesterol 42mg • Sodium 407 mg • Fiber 2g

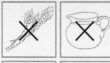

SCONES WITHOUT EGGS

Makes 8 scones

If you want this to be a sweeter scone, increase the sugar to ¼ cup. Use this recipe to make egg-free versions of the other scones in this chapter.

¼ cup (½ stick) butter or margarine
¾ cup 2% milk (cow, rice, or soy)
1¼ cups sorghum flour
½ cup tapioca flour
2 tablespoons granulated sugar or fructose powder

1½ teaspoons cream of tartar
1 teaspoon xanthan gum
¾ teaspoon baking soda
½ teaspoon salt
¼ teaspoon soy lecithin
½ cup currants (optional)

1. Preheat oven to 425°F. Grease nonstick baking sheet or line with parchment paper.
2. In food processor, blend butter, milk, flours, sugar or fructose powder, cream of tartar, xanthan gum, baking soda, salt, and lecithin. Process just until mixed. Add currants (if using) and pulse a few times to incorporate. Work quickly so the leavening doesn't lose its power. Dough will be soft.
3. Transfer dough to prepared baking sheet, patting with spatula into 8-inch circle, ¾-inch thick. Bake for 15–20 minutes, or until deeply browned. For crispier, wedge-shaped pieces, cut into 8 wedges and return to oven for the final 5 minutes of baking.

Nutrition Information (per scone)
Calories 220 • Fat 8g • Protein 7g • Carbohydrates 33g • Cholesterol 16mg • Sodium 300mg • Fiber 3g

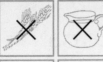 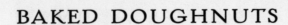

BAKED DOUGHNUTS

Makes 12 doughnuts

These are an alternative to traditional fried doughnuts.

2 cups Flour Blend (page 276)

2 teaspoons xanthan gum

1½ teaspoons baking powder

1½ teaspoons baking soda

1 teaspoon unflavored gelatin powder

½ teaspoon salt

2 teaspoons ground cinnamon

¼ teaspoon ground cloves

¼ teaspoon ground nutmeg

1 large egg, or ¼ cup soft silken tofu

⅔ cup packed light brown sugar or maple sugar

½ cup frozen apple-juice concentrate, thawed

½ cup drained applesauce

½ cup maple syrup

3 tablespoons canola oil

1. Preheat oven to 375°F. Grease molds of mini-Bundt or mini-angel food cake tins (or use two 6-cup muffin or cupcake tins).

2. In large mixer bowl, add flours, xanthan gum, baking powder, baking soda, gelatin powder, salt, cinnamon, cloves, and nutmeg and stir to blend. In another bowl, with electric mixer, combine egg, brown sugar, apple-juice concentrate, applesauce, maple syrup, and oil until thoroughly blended.

3. Divide the batter in half since you'll bake batter in two batches. Spoon half of batter into prepared mini-molds—about 2 generous tablespoons per mold. (If using muffin tins, fill each two-thirds full.)

4. Bake for 20–25 minutes or until tops spring back when touched lightly. Loosen edges of doughnuts with sharp knife and turn out onto wire rack to cool. Clean pan, grease again, and fill molds with 2 tablespoons batter each. Bake for 20–25 minutes.

Nutrition Information (per doughnut)
Calories 240 • Fat 5g • Protein 4g • Carbohydrates 49g • Cholesterol 15mg • Sodium 307mg • Fiber 0.5g

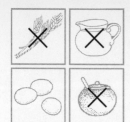

BANANA BREAD

Serves 12

Wait—don't throw out those overripe bananas. Freeze them for use later in this delicious recipe. For an egg-free version, see page 56.

⅔ cup packed light brown sugar or
   maple sugar*

2 large eggs

3 tablespoons canola oil

1 teaspoon vanilla extract

1¾ cups Flour Blend (page 276)

½ teaspoon xanthan gum

½ teaspoon salt

2 teaspoons baking powder

1 teaspoon ground cinnamon

⅛ teaspoon *each* ground cardamom
   and mace (optional)

1½ cups mashed ripe bananas

½ cup chopped nuts of your choice
   (optional)

½ cup raisins (optional)

1. Preheat oven to 350°F. Grease one 9x5-inch nonstick loaf pan. For smaller loaves that bake more thoroughly, use three 5x3-inch nonstick loaf pans.

2. Cream sugar, eggs, oil, and vanilla with electric mixer in medium mixer bowl. Mix together flours, xanthan gum, salt, baking powder, and spices in separate bowl. Add flour mixture to egg mixture, alternating with bananas. Stir in nuts and raisins (if using). Batter will be soft.

3. Pour batter into prepared pan(s). Bake large loaf for 1 hour; small loaves for 45 minutes. Cool thoroughly on wire rack before cutting.

Nutrition Information (per serving)

Calories 240 • Fat 6g • Protein 3g • Carbohydrates 47g • Cholesterol 30mg • Sodium 160mg • Fiber 1.5g

*Sugar Alternative: Use ⅓ cup pure maple syrup in place of ⅔ cup brown sugar. You will need to add ⅛ teaspoon baking soda.

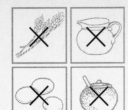

BANANA BREAD
WITHOUT EGGS

Serves 12

This bread is the perfect way to use up those overripe bananas. It will be a little heavier than the version made with eggs.

1 cup mashed ripe bananas	2½ teaspoons baking powder
⅓ cup honey or maple syrup	½ teaspoon xanthan gum
⅓ cup 2% milk (cow, rice, or soy)	½ teaspoon salt
3 tablespoons canola oil	¼ teaspoon soy lecithin
1 teaspoon vanilla extract	1¼ teaspoons ground cinnamon
1 teaspoon molasses or maple syrup	⅛ teaspoon ground cardamom (optional)
¾ cup potato starch	⅛ teaspoon ground mace (optional)
½ cup sorghum flour	½ cup dark raisins or currants (optional)
½ cup garbanzo/fava bean flour	½ cup chopped pecans or walnuts (optional)

1. Preheat oven to 350°F. Grease three 5x3-inch nonstick loaf pans or one 9x5-inch nonstick loaf pan. (Bread bakes more thoroughly in smaller pans.)
2. In large mixer bowl with electric mixer, cream mashed bananas, honey, milk, oil, vanilla, and molasses until thoroughly blended. Add flours, baking powder, xanthan gum, salt, lecithin, cinnamon, and the other spices (if using) and mix together thoroughly. Stir in raisins and nuts (if using). Batter will be somewhat soft. Spoon batter into prepared pan(s) and smooth top of batter with spatula.
3. Bake small loaves for 35–40 minutes, large loaf for 50–60 minutes, or until tops are golden brown. Cool on wire rack. Slice with serrated knife or electric knife when cool.

Nutrition Information (per serving)
Calories 200 • Fat 6g • Protein 3g • Carbohydrates 33g • Cholesterol 1mg • Sodium 175mg • Fiber 1.5g

Note: If raisins and nuts are omitted, use two instead of three 5x3-inch loaf pans because the volume of the bread is considerably reduced. Banana bread without nuts and raisins may be somewhat gummier; baking in smaller pans will help reduce this problem.

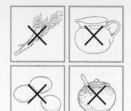

BLUEBERRY-LEMON BREAD

Serves 12

Serve this delectable quick bread while it's still warm, slathered with your favorite spread.

2⅓ cups Flour Blend (page 276)	¼ teaspoon soy lecithin
1½ teaspoons xanthan gum	¼ cup canola oil
2½ teaspoons baking powder	2 large eggs,* or ½ cup soft silken tofu
1 teaspoon unflavored gelatin powder	1 teaspoon vanilla extract
1 teaspoon salt	1 cup 2% milk (cow, rice, or soy)
⅓ cup granulated sugar or fructose powder	Grated zest from 1 lemon
	1¼ cups fresh or frozen blueberries

1. Preheat oven to 375°F. Grease three 5x3-inch nonstick loaf pans.
2. In large bowl, combine dry ingredients. With electric mixer, blend in oil, eggs, vanilla, milk, and lemon zest until very smooth. Gently stir in blueberries.
3. Spoon dough into prepared pans. Bake for 25–30 minutes (add 5 minutes if using frozen blueberries), or until tops are lightly browned. Remove from oven.

Nutrition Information (per slice)
Calories 250 • Fat 6g • Protein 3g • Carbohydrates 48g • Cholesterol 32mg • Sodium 275mg • Fiber 1g

Cranberry-Orange Bread: Add 1 tablespoon grated orange zest and 1¼ cups chopped cranberries.

*Egg Alternative: You can also use ½ cup flaxseed mixture (see page 108). Increase baking powder to 1 tablespoon. Reduce oil by 1 tablespoon. Bake for 5 minutes longer. Bread will be heavy and dense without eggs and somewhat darker due to the flaxseed.

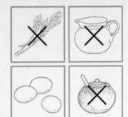

SALLY LUNN (SOLEIL ET LUNE) BREAD

Serves 12

Serve this bread with a dusting of powdered sugar or with orange marmalade. If you wish, assemble the dough the night before and let rise, covered, in refrigerator all night. The next morning, remove from refrigerator and bake for an extra 10 minutes, or until done. Because eggs provide part of the leavening, this is not an egg-free bread.

BREAD

1 tablespoon active dry yeast

¼ cup granulated sugar or fructose powder, divided

½ cup warm water (110°F)

3½ cups Flour Blend (page 276)

2 teaspoons xanthan gum

1¼ teaspoons salt

1 teaspoon unflavored gelatin powder

¾ teaspoon ground mace

1½ tablespoons grated orange zest

1 cup hot orange juice (115°F)

⅓ cup butter or margarine, or ¼ cup canola oil

3 large eggs, at room temperature

3 teaspoons vanilla extract

GLAZE

3 tablespoons fresh orange juice

3 tablespoons powdered sugar or fructose powder

2 tablespoons grated orange zest

1. Dissolve yeast and 1 teaspoon of the sugar or fructose powder in warm water and set aside until foamy, about 5 minutes.
2. Combine flours, remaining sugar or fructose powder, xanthan gum, salt, gelatin, and mace in large mixer bowl with electric mixer. Add orange zest, orange juice, butter or canola oil, eggs, vanilla, and yeast mixture. Beat with regular beaters 2 minutes. Batter will be very soft and sticky.
3. Grease 10-inch nonstick Bundt pan. Add dough to prepared pan. Cover loosely with oiled plastic wrap; let rise at room temperature (75–80°F) for 45 minutes–1 hour, until doubled in bulk.

4. Ten minutes before baking, preheat oven to 350°F. Remove plastic wrap and bake bread for 30–35 minutes, until wooden pick inserted into center comes out clean. Let cool for 5 minutes in pan, then unmold bread and place on wire rack to cool.

5. In small saucepan or in microwave oven, heat orange juice, sugar, and orange zest until sugar melts. Brush warm bread with glaze.

Nutrition Information (per serving)
Calories 300 • Fat 3g • Protein 4g • Carbohydrates 69g • Cholesterol 46mg • Sodium 260mg • Fiber 1g

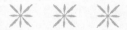

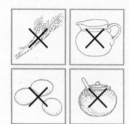

RAISIN BREAD

Serves 12

I like this bread for breakfast, toasted nicely and brushed with a bit of margarine.

2¼ teaspoons active dry yeast
¼ cup packed light brown sugar or maple sugar
1 cup warm water (110°F)
2 cups + 1 tablespoon Flour Blend (page 276)
⅓ cup dry milk powder or nondairy milk powder
1½ teaspoons xanthan gum

1 teaspoon unflavored gelatin powder
1 teaspoon salt
1 teaspoon ground cinnamon
¼ teaspoon soy lecithin (optional)
2 large eggs, at room temperature, or ½ cup Flax Mix (page 108)
¼ cup canola oil
1 teaspoon vinegar
½ cup dark raisins or currants

HAND:

1. Have ingredients at room temperature for best rising. Combine yeast and 2 teaspoons of brown sugar in warm water and let foam 5 minutes.

2. In large mixer bowl using regular beaters (not dough hooks), combine flours, milk powder, xanthan gum, gelatin, salt, remaining brown sugar, cinnamon, and lecithin (if using). Add eggs, oil, vinegar, and yeast mixture.

3. Blend ingredients on low until liquid is incorporated, then increase mixer speed to high and beat 1 minute. Scrape sides of bowl occasionally with spatula. Stir in raisins or currants.

4. For smaller loaves, grease three 5x3-inch nonstick loaf pans. Divide dough among prepared pans, smooth tops with spatula, and put in warm place to rise for 35–40 minutes, until doubled in bulk. For one large loaf, grease a 9x5-inch nonstick loaf pan. Place dough in pan, smooth top with spatula, and let dough rise in warm place for 35–40 minutes, until doubled in bulk.

5. Preheat oven to 350°F. Bake small loaves for 20–25 minutes, large loaf for 45 minutes. Let cool for 5 minutes; remove from pan. Cool on wire rack.

MACHINE:

Spray pan with cooking spray. Add room temperature ingredients in order listed by manufacturer. Set controls and bake. Makes a 1-pound loaf. (Loaf will be heavier and denser if using flaxseed.)

Nutrition Information (per serving)
Calories 275 • Fat 11g • Protein 4g • Carbohydrates 44g • Cholesterol 30mg • Sodium 200mg • Fiber 1g

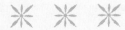

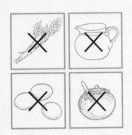

BLUEBERRY-APRICOT COFFEE CAKE

Serves 12

This is a great breakfast dish. You can make it ahead, freeze it, and then thaw it at room temperature. Heat gently just before serving. You can find the rolled rice flakes for this recipe in natural food stores or from www.vitamincottage.com or www.enjoylifefoods.com.

CAKE

⅓ cup butter or margarine, or ¼ cup canola oil

¾ cup granulated sugar or fructose powder

2 large eggs*

1 tablespoon grated orange zest

1½ cups Flour Blend (page 276)

1 teaspoon xanthan gum

½ teaspoon baking powder

½ teaspoon baking soda

½ teaspoon salt

½ cup + 2 tablespoons 2% milk (cow, rice, or soy)

2 tablespoons vinegar

1 teaspoon vanilla extract

½ cup dried blueberries

½ cup chopped dried apricots

TOPPING

¼ cup packed light brown sugar or maple sugar

½ teaspoon ground cinnamon

¼ teaspoon ground nutmeg

2 tablespoons canola oil

2 tablespoons brown rice flour

¼ cup chopped nuts of choice

¼ cup rolled rice flakes

1. Preheat oven to 350°F. Grease 11x7-inch nonstick baking pan.
2. Using electric mixer and large mixer bowl, cream butter, sugar, eggs, and orange zest on medium speed until smooth.
3. In medium mixer bowl, combine flours, xanthan gum, baking powder, baking soda, and salt. In another medium mixer bowl, combine milk, vinegar, and vanilla.
4. On low speed, beat dry ingredients into egg mixture, alternating with milk mixture, beginning and ending with dry ingredients. Mix just until combined. Stir in blueberries and apricots.
5. Spoon batter into prepared pan. Mix topping ingredients and sprinkle on top. Bake for 35 minutes, until top is golden brown and wooden pick inserted in center comes out clean.

Nutrition Information (per serving)
Calories 350 • Fat 11g • Protein 4g • Carbohydrates 62g • Cholesterol 50mg • Sodium 257mg • Fiber 1g

*Egg Alternative: Omit eggs. Use ½ cup soft silken tofu. Increase baking powder and baking soda by ⅛ teaspoon each. Cake will be heavier and denser.

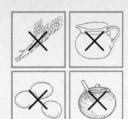

CAFFEE BORGIA
COFFEE CAKE

Serves 12

Borrowed from the chocolate-infused coffee drink that is also flavored with orange, this cake is perfect for brunch. If you're a coffee lover, be sure to try this one.

CAKE

¾ cup packed light brown sugar
  or maple sugar

¼ cup canola oil

2 large eggs, or ½ cup soft silken tofu

2 tablespoons grated orange zest

2 teaspoons vanilla extract

½ cup warm brewed coffee (110°F)

1½ cups Flour Blend (page 276)

1 tablespoon unsweetened cocoa
  powder (not Dutch process)

1 tablespoon espresso powder, or 2
  tablespoons instant coffee granules

2¼ teaspoons baking powder

1 teaspoon ground cinnamon

½ teaspoon xanthan gum

½ teaspoon salt

TOPPING

¼ cup packed light brown sugar
  or maple sugar

2 tablespoons brown rice flour

1 teaspoon unsweetened cocoa
  powder

1 teaspoon ground cinnamon

1 tablespoon canola oil

1. Preheat oven to 350°F. Grease 8-inch square nonstick baking pan.
2. Using electric mixer and large mixer bowl, cream sugar, oil, eggs or tofu, orange zest, and vanilla. Add coffee and blend on medium speed about 1 minute, until very smooth. Add remaining cake ingredients and mix just until combined. Pour batter into prepared pan.
3. To make topping, combine ingredients thoroughly with pastry blender or fork. Sprinkle topping on batter. Bake for 25–30 minutes, until wooden pick inserted in center comes out clean. Cool before cutting.

Nutrition Information (per serving made with eggs)
Calories 290 • Fat 11g • Protein 3g • Carbohydrates 48g • Cholesterol 36mg • Sodium 205mg • Fiber 1g

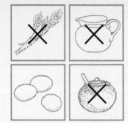

PANCAKES

Makes eight 4-inch pancakes (Serves 4)

Make these pancakes for your family on the weekends so you can savor them over coffee while you plan your day.

1 large egg

½ cup plain nonfat yogurt, or ½ cup
   2% milk (cow, rice, or soy)

½ cup Flour Blend (page 276)

1 teaspoon granulated sugar or
   fructose powder

1 teaspoon baking powder

½ teaspoon baking soda

½ teaspoon salt

1 tablespoon canola oil

1 teaspoon vanilla extract

Additional canola oil, for frying

1. Blend egg and yogurt in blender or whisk vigorously in bowl. Add remaining ingredients and blend thoroughly.
2. Heat additional oil in large, nonstick skillet or grill over medium heat. Pour a scant ¼ cup of batter into skillet and cook 3–5 minutes, until tops are bubbly. Turn and cook 2–3 minutes, until golden brown.

Nutrition Information (per 2-pancake serving)
Calories 170 • Fat 6g • Protein 3g • Carbohydrates 28g • Cholesterol 49mg • Sodium 541mg •
   Fiber 0.5g

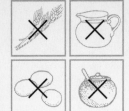

PANCAKES WITHOUT EGGS

Makes eight 4-inch pancakes (Serves 4)

⅔ cup 2% milk (cow, rice, or soy)

2 teaspoons egg replacer powder

½ cup + 1 tablespoon Flour Blend (page 276)

1 teaspoon granulated sugar or fructose powder

¾ teaspoon baking soda

½ teaspoon salt

1 teaspoon vanilla extract

1 tablespoon canola oil

Additional canola oil, for frying

1. Blend milk and egg replacer in blender 1 minute, then blend in remaining ingredients.
2. Heat additional oil in large, nonstick skillet or grill over medium heat. For each pancake, pour 3 tablespoons batter into skillet and cook 2–3 minutes, until tops are bubbly. Turn; cook 1–2 minutes, until golden brown.

Nutrition Information (per 2-pancake serving)
Calories 170 • Fat 5g • Protein 3g • Carbohydrates 32g • Cholesterol 3mg • Sodium 636mg • Fiber 0.5g

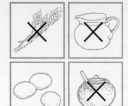

WAFFLES

Makes four 8-inch waffles (Serves 8, ½ waffle each)

This waffle recipe is easy and dependable. See egg-free version on page 66.

1¾ cups Flour Blend (page 276)	2 large eggs
1 tablespoon granulated sugar or fructose powder	2 tablespoons canola oil
2 teaspoons baking powder	2 tablespoons vinegar
½ teaspoon salt	1⅓ cups 2% milk (cow, rice, or soy)
	1 teaspoon vanilla extract

1. Combine dry ingredients in medium mixer bowl. In separate mixer bowl, whisk together eggs, oil, vinegar, milk, and vanilla. Whisk liquid mixture into flour mixture until thoroughly combined.
2. Preheat waffle iron. Cook on waffle iron according to manufacturer's instructions.

Nutrition Information (per ½ waffle)
Calories 280 • Fat 8g • Protein 4g • Carbohydrates 48g • Cholesterol 48mg • Sodium 410mg • Fiber 0.5g

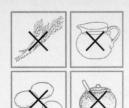

WAFFLES WITHOUT EGGS

Makes four 8-inch waffles (Serves 8, ½ waffle each)

Even without eggs, these waffles are crisp and delicious.

1¾ cups Flour Blend (page 276)
1 tablespoon granulated sugar or
  fructose powder
1 teaspoon baking soda
½ teaspoon salt
½ teaspoon xanthan gum

2 tablespoons canola oil
1¼ cups buttermilk, or 1 tablespoon
  vinegar or lemon juice with enough
  2% milk (cow, rice, or soy) to equal
  1¼ cups
1 teaspoon vanilla extract

1. In small mixer bowl, mix together flours, sugar, baking soda, salt, and xanthan gum. Whisk in oil, buttermilk or vinegar mixture, and vanilla.
2. Heat waffle iron. Pour ¼ of batter onto heated waffle iron. Follow manufacturer's directions for your waffle iron. Close and bake about 4–6 minutes, until steaming stops. Repeat with remaining batter.

Nutrition Information (per ½ waffle)
Calories 230 • Fat 4.5g • Protein 3g • Carbohydrates 48g • Cholesterol 1mg • Sodium 464mg • Fiber 0.5g

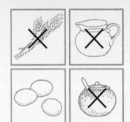

EGGS BENEDICT

Serves 4

You may omit the eggs in this recipe and replace them with poached vegetables such as asparagus, broccoli, or spinach.

1⅓ cups Hollandaise Sauce (page 68)
4 English Muffins (page 44)
8 pieces Canadian-style bacon, thinly
   sliced
8 large eggs, poached

Paprika, for garnish
¼ cup fresh chopped parsley, or 2
   tablespoons dried parsley, for
   garnish

1. Prepare Hollandaise sauce according to recipe and keep warm in double boiler.
2. Warm sliced English muffins in microwave or wrapped in foil in a 250°F oven.
3. Meanwhile, warm Canadian-style bacon in microwave to desired serving temperature.
4. Arrange two halves of English muffin on each of 4 plates. Top each half with slice of Canadian-style bacon, then poached egg. Top with Hollandaise sauce. Garnish with paprika and parsley.

Nutrition Information (per serving)
Calories 525 • Fat 27g • Protein 40g • Carbohydrates 44g • Cholesterol 570mg • Sodium 1,808mg
   • Fiber 2g

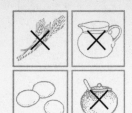

HOLLANDAISE SAUCE

Makes 1 cup (Serves 4)

This delightfully creamy sauce contains eggs.

2 large egg yolks
1 cup Yogurt Cheese (page 114) or
   soft silken tofu
3 tablespoons fresh lemon
   juice
½ teaspoon xanthan gum

2 tablespoons butter, margarine,
   or canola oil
¼ teaspoon salt
¼ teaspoon dry mustard
⅛ teaspoon cayenne pepper
⅛ teaspoon white pepper

1. Blend egg yolks, yogurt cheese or silken tofu, lemon juice, and xanthan gum in blender until light and fluffy. Place egg yolk mixture in top of double boiler set over simmering, not boiling, water. Don't let bottom of double boiler touch water. Add butter, whisking constantly until mixture thickens. If too thick, add 1 tablespoon or more of hot water.
2. Remove sauce from heat and stir in remaining ingredients. Hollandaise mixture can be kept warm over simmering water for about 30 minutes. If it starts to separate, add 1 teaspoon of boiling water and whisk briskly until smooth.

Nutrition Information (per ¼-cup serving)
Calories 125 • Fat 11g • Protein 5g • Carbohydrates 6g • Cholesterol 120mg • Sodium 240mg • Fiber 0g

Note: You can make your own dry mustard by grinding mustard seeds in a small coffee grinder.

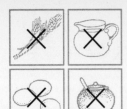

BREAKFAST SAUSAGE

Serves 12

If you love sausage in the "wurst" way, this recipe makes it easy to include the flavorful meat on your breakfast plate. If you want an even lower fat content, try using half ground turkey and half ground pork. You can either shape the meat into patties or links—or brown the meat in a crumbled fashion. You can sprinkle the crumbles onto your scrambled eggs or your favorite pizza. Yum!

1 pound ground pork, turkey, or beef	½ teaspoon black pepper
1 teaspoon rubbed sage	½ teaspoon fennel seeds
½ teaspoon salt	¼ teaspoon ground nutmeg
½ teaspoon dried thyme leaves	⅛ teaspoon ground cloves
½ teaspoon ground cumin	⅛ teaspoon cayenne pepper
½ teaspoon dried savory leaves	

1. Blend all ingredients together in large mixer bowl using your hands or large spatula. Form into 12 patties or links (spray hands with cooking spray first).
2. Preheat nonstick skillet. Fry sausages over medium heat until cooked through. Or simply crumble mixture in skillet and brown.

Nutrition Information (per serving)
Calories 110 • Fat 8g • Protein 10g • Carbohydrates 1g • Cholesterol 36mg • Sodium 125mg • Fiber 0.5g

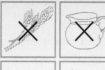

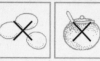

BREAKFAST FRUIT PIZZA

Makes 6 slices

Surprise your children or your guests with this unique pizza.

PIZZA

1 tablespoon active dry yeast

⅔ cup brown rice flour or
   sorghum flour

½ cup tapioca flour

2 teaspoons xanthan gum

½ teaspoon salt

1 teaspoon ground cinnamon

1 teaspoon unflavored gelatin
   powder

¼ teaspoon ground mace (optional)

¾ cup warm 2% milk (cow, rice,
   or soy) (110°F)

1 tablespoon granulated sugar or
   fructose powder

1 teaspoon canola oil

1 teaspoon cider vinegar

2 teaspoons grated lemon zest

Rice flour

TOPPING

½ cup fresh orange juice

2 tablespoons granulated sugar
   or fructose powder

1 tablespoon cornstarch

¼ teaspoon ground cinnamon

¼ teaspoon salt

2 cups finely chopped fruit:
   apples, peaches, plums,
   blueberries, etc., or use dried fruit:
   cherries, cranberries, apricots

1 cup chopped nuts of your choice
   (optional)

PIZZA:

1. Preheat oven to 425°F. Grease 12-inch nonstick pizza pan.
2. In medium mixer bowl using regular beaters, blend yeast, flours, xanthan gum, salt, cinnamon, gelatin powder, and mace (if using) on low speed. Add warm milk, sugar or fructose powder, oil, vinegar, and lemon zest.
3. Beat on high speed for 2 minutes. Dough will resemble soft bread dough. Put mixture onto prepared pan. Liberally sprinkle rice flour onto dough; then press dough into pan, continuing to sprinkle dough with flour to prevent sticking. Make edges thicker to hold toppings. Bake crust for 10 minutes. Remove from oven.

TOPPING:

1. Combine orange juice, sugar, cornstarch, cinnamon, and salt in small saucepan and cook over low-medium heat, continuing to stir until mixture thickens. Stir in fruit. Spread filling on baked pizza crust.
2. Return pizza to oven and bake for another 10–15 minutes, or until golden brown. Add nuts (if using) during the final 5 minutes of baking. Cool for 5 minutes before serving.

Nutrition Information (per slice)

Calories 320 • Fat 14g • Protein 7g • Carbohydrates 47g • Cholesterol 1mg • Sodium 320mg • Fiber 5g

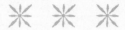

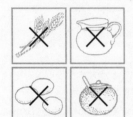

BIRCHER-MUESLI

Makes 8 cups

I've always loved this cereal and now I have it frequently at home, knowing it contains no wheat or gluten. You can assemble the rolled rice flakes, nuts, and spices the night before. Then add the fresh fruit and yogurt (or milk) just before serving. For a large family, double this recipe. I've enjoyed this wonderful breakfast dish both cold and warm.

2 cups rolled rice flakes
2 teaspoons grated lemon zest
1 tablespoon grated orange zest
1 cup fresh orange juice
½ teaspoon ground cinnamon
¼ cup dried tart cherries
¼ cup golden raisins
¼ cup dried apricots

¼ cup dried blueberries
½ cup coarsely chopped nuts
  of your choice
1 apple, finely chopped
1 pear, finely chopped
1 banana, finely chopped
1 cup yogurt, or ¾ cup 2% milk
  (cow, rice, or soy)

Combine all ingredients in large serving bowl. Serve chilled or heat to desired temperature in saucepan. If mixture is too thick, add additional yogurt or milk to achieve desired consistency. You can find the rolled rice flakes for this recipe in natural food stores or from www.vitamincottage.com or www.enjoylifefoods.com.

Nutrition Information (per cup)
Calories 210 • Fat 6g • Protein 4g • Carbohydrates 40g • Cholesterol 0mg • Sodium 75mg • Fiber 3g

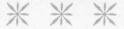

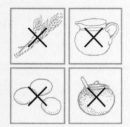

GOURMET GRANOLA

Makes 4 cups (8 servings)

This makes a small quantity, but it is enough to make a fairly thin layer on a 15x10-inch jelly-roll pan. If you have a very large oven and/or very large baking pans, you can double the recipe. For lower-fat version, omit canola oil and spray mix with cooking spray each time you stir during browning process described below. Also, the sweetener you use will affect the flavor somewhat. You can vary the dried fruit as you wish. In fact, dried blueberries or dried peaches will also work nicely.

2 cups rolled rice flakes
½ teaspoon ground cinnamon
¼ cup sesame seeds
¼ cup sunflower or pumpkin seeds
¼ cup almond slivers
¼ cup unsweetened coconut flakes
1 teaspoon vanilla extract

2 teaspoons canola oil
¼ teaspoon salt
¼ cup honey or agave nectar
¼ cup golden raisins
¼ cup dried cranberries
¼ cup chopped dried apricots

1. Combine all ingredients except raisins, cranberries, and apricots in large plastic container with tight-fitting lid or in large plastic bag. Shake until well mixed.
2. Grease baking sheet and spread granola on prepared sheet. Bake for 30–40 minutes at 300°F, or until lightly browned. Stir every 10 minutes to assure even browning. Remove from oven and let cool for 15 minutes. Add dried fruit. Cool completely. Store in airtight container in a dark, dry place.

Nutrition Information (per serving)

Calories 210 • Fat 9g • Protein 4g • Carbohydrates 31g • Cholesterol 1mg • Sodium 128mg • Fiber 3g

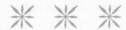

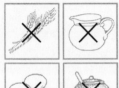

GRANOLA BARS

Makes 18 bars

You can vary the fruits in this easy but highly nutritious granola bar. For example, dried blueberries or cranberries also work great. The potato flour (not potato starch) gives the bars a nice, chewy texture that more closely resembles granola bars made with oatmeal. A food processor is especially useful for this recipe because it chops ingredients evenly, making for a more consistent granola bar. The bars will be thin. Rolled rice cakes are available at www.vitamincottage.com or www.enjoylifefoods.com.

¼ cup applesauce	1 teaspoon vanilla extract
¼ cup honey or agave nectar	2 teaspoons canola oil
¼ cup golden raisins	¼ cup potato flour (not potato starch)
¼ cup dried tart cherries	2 cups rolled rice flakes
¼ cup chopped dried apricots	1 teaspoon xanthan gum
1 tablespoon grated orange zest	1 teaspoon ground cinnamon

1 teaspoon baking powder
¼ cup sesame seeds
¼ cup shelled sunflower or pumpkin
  seeds

¼ cup almond slivers
¼ cup unsweetened coconut flakes
½ teaspoon salt

1. Preheat oven to 325°F. Grease 13x9-inch nonstick baking pan and line with waxed paper or parchment paper if you plan to invert pan. Grease again and set aside.
2. Combine all ingredients in food processor. Process until mixture is thoroughly combined.
3. Spread batter evenly in prepared pan. Bake for 30–35 minutes, or until mixture begins to brown around edges. Remove from oven and let cool for 10 minutes. If inverting pan onto a cutting surface, do so now. Otherwise, let bars cool to room temperature before cutting.

Nutrition Information (per bar)
Calories 100 • Fat 4g • Protein 2g • Carbohydrates 15g • Cholesterol 1mg • Sodium 117mg • Fiber 2g

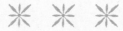

HOT BREAKFAST CEREAL

For many of us, hot cereal is an absolute necessity at breakfast—summer, winter, spring, or fall. Just because you don't eat wheat or gluten doesn't mean you can't have cooked cereal. There are many other grains to cook for breakfast besides wheat or oatmeal.

Many stores carry quick-cooking versions of some cereals such as buckwheat or rice. And Bob's Red Mill Natural Foods has a new gluten-free multigrain hot cereal (see Resources). If you want to "speed up" the cooking process of larger whole grains (such as brown rice or buckwheat), try whirling them in a blender first. This breaks down the fiber a bit, allowing the grains to cook more quickly.

GRAIN (1 CUP)	WATER	APPROXIMATE COOKING TIME
Amaranth	2 cups	20–25 minutes
Brown rice	2½ cups	50–55 minutes
Buckwheat	2 cups	15–20 minutes
Millet	2½ cups	35–45 minutes
Polenta (corn) grits	4 cups	10 minutes
Quinoa	2 cups	15–20 minutes
Sorghum (milo)	2 cups	20–25 minutes
(soak overnight beforehand)		*(let stand 5 minutes)*
White rice	2 cups	20 minutes
Wild rice	4 cups	40 minutes

APPETIZERS & SNACKS

Appetizers are designed to take the edge off hunger or to whet the appetite for the main course. Sometimes, appetizers can be a meal in themselves. You'll find a wide range of tasty tidbits here that everyone will enjoy—even if they can't eat wheat, dairy, eggs, or cane sugar.

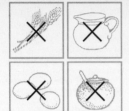

APPETIZER MEATBALLS

Serves 12 (3 meatballs each)

I like to use this recipe when I want something hot on the buffet table, yet I can prepare it ahead of time. A chafing dish works just great, but I've also served the meatballs in a slow cooker. Double the recipe for larger groups.

MEATBALLS

1 pound lean ground beef

½ cup crushed gluten-free cornflakes
   or gluten-free cracker crumbs

¼ cup finely chopped onion

2 tablespoons ketchup

1 teaspoon dried thyme leaves

1 teaspoon salt

¼ teaspoon black pepper

¼ teaspoon chili powder

SAUCE

1 can (8 ounces) tomato sauce

¼ cup ketchup

2 tablespoons sweet pickle relish

2 tablespoons finely chopped onion

2 tablespoons light brown sugar or
   maple sugar

1 tablespoon vinegar

1 tablespoon Lea & Perrins
   Worcestershire sauce

½ teaspoon salt

¼ teaspoon black pepper

¼ teaspoon ground allspice

¼ cup water

1. Preheat oven to 400°F. Grease baking sheet or line with parchment paper.
2. In large bowl, combine beef, cornflakes, onion, ketchup, thyme, salt, pepper, and chili powder until well mixed. Shape into 36 meatballs (about 1 tablespoon each). Place on prepared baking sheet. Bake for 15–20 minutes, until nicely browned.
3. Meanwhile, in medium saucepan, combine tomato sauce, ketchup, pickle relish, tomato sauce, onion, sugar, vinegar, Worcestershire sauce, salt, pepper, allspice, and water. Bring to boiling, lower heat, and simmer for 15 minutes. Add meatballs and simmer another 15 minutes. Spear meatballs with wooden picks.

Nutrition Information (per serving)
Calories 100 • Fat 4g • Protein 8g • Carbohydrates 9g • Cholesterol 14mg • Sodium 470mg • Fiber 1g

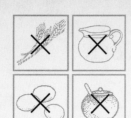

BUFFALO WINGS

Serves 16

You can eat these tasty wings plain or dip in your favorite dipping sauce. Have plenty of napkins handy. These wings are a little bit messy—but definitely worth it!

4 pounds chicken wings
  or drummettes
1 tablespoon olive oil
1 tablespoon paprika
2 teaspoons celery salt
1 teaspoon garlic powder
1 teaspoon onion powder

1 teaspoon granulated sugar
  or fructose powder
1 teaspoon dried oregano leaves
1 teaspoon dried thyme leaves
1 teaspoon dry mustard
1 teaspoon ground white pepper
½ teaspoon cayenne pepper

1. Wash and pat the chicken dry with paper towels. If using whole chicken wings, cut off wings at first joint and reserve discarded pieces for another use (such as chicken stock).
2. In large bowl or plastic freezer bag, toss wings with olive oil. Combine remaining ingredients. Then toss wings with spice mixture until thoroughly coated.
3. Refrigerate at least 2 hours or overnight. Arrange wings in shallow baking pan or on baking sheet. Preheat oven to 450°F. Bake wings for 12–15 minutes on middle rack of oven. Turn wings and continue baking for another 12–15 minutes, until crispy. As an alternative, you may grill wings on barbecue grill until done. Serve with dipping sauce of your choice.

Nutrition Information (per serving)
Calories 300 • Fat 20g • Protein 26g • Carbohydrates 1g • Cholesterol 79mg • Sodium 77mg • Fiber 0.5g

Note: You can make your own dry mustard by grinding mustard seeds in a small coffee grinder.

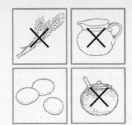

CHICKEN FINGERS

Serves 4 (½ breast each)

Kids love this easy-to-make dish. You can bake a bunch and freeze them. They make great snacks for after-school treats.

    4 boneless, skinless chicken breast halves
    1 egg, beaten
    ½ cup 2% milk (cow, rice, or soy)
    Breading Mix (page 118)
    ¼ cup canola oil, for frying
    Salt
    Pepper

1. Slice each chicken breast diagonally into ½-inch-wide strips. Whisk together egg and milk in bowl. Dip each strip into egg mixture, then into breading mix.
2. Heat oil in deep pan or skillet. Fry chicken fingers in oil until browned, turning to promote even browning. Add salt and pepper to taste. Or bake on nonstick baking sheet at 350°F for 30 minutes, until nicely browned.

Nutrition Information (per serving)
Calories 270 • Fat 16g • Protein 28g • Carbohydrates 1g • Cholesterol 110mg • Sodium 90mg •
    Fiber 1g

Egg-free Chicken Fingers: Omit egg and dip chicken in milk only. Bake as directed.

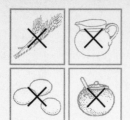

MINIATURE CHICKEN OR TUNA SALAD FOCACCIA SANDWICHES

Makes 20 sandwiches (Serves 10, 2 sandwiches each)

Focaccia makes extremely flavorful sandwiches and is so simple to prepare. Choose from this wide variety of savory fillings to spread between pieces of the focaccia. If you are making them for a party, arrange decoratively on a large platter garnished with sprigs of fresh parsley or your favorite herbs.

2 cups ground cooked chicken (about 2 whole chicken breasts), or 2 cups low-salt canned tuna (about 4 small cans)

½ cup Homemade Mayonnaise (page 115)

1 teaspoon dried thyme leaves

1 teaspoon dried dill weed

1 teaspoon onion powder

½ teaspoon celery salt

¼ teaspoon black pepper

Focaccia (page 23)

Fresh parsley or herbs, for garnish (optional)

1. Combine all chicken or tuna salad ingredients in bowl and mash together with fork. Chill until serving time.
2. Cut focaccia into 20 equal pieces. Using sharp, serrated knife, carefully slice each piece horizontally. Spread 2 tablespoons of filling between 2 slices. Garnish with fresh parsley or herbs and serve immediately or cover tightly and refrigerate up to 4 hours.

Nutrition Information (for filling for 2 sandwiches)*
Calories 135 • Fat 8g • Protein 6g • Carbohydrates 10g • Cholesterol 34mg • Sodium 205mg • Fiber 0.5g

*For Nutrition Information for Focaccia, see page 23.

ADDITIONAL FILLINGS
* Thinly sliced cucumber, red onion, Ranch Dressing (page 95), and lettuce.
* Paper-thin slices of prosciutto and Granny Smith apples, fresh basil leaves, mayonnaise, and lettuce.
* Softened goat cheese (or creamed tofu) with raisins, orange marmalade, whole mint leaves, and lettuce. (Goat cheese is not dairy-free.)

- Paper-thin slices of roast beef and red onion, gluten-free horseradish sauce, butter or margarine, and lettuce.
- Thinly sliced plum tomatoes, red onion, guacamole dip, and lettuce.
- Thinly sliced smoked turkey, red onion, Dijon mustard, and lettuce.
- Paper-thin slices of smoked ham, hummus, and lettuce.
- Crumbled crisp bacon, finely chopped oven-dried tomatoes, and lettuce.

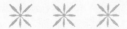

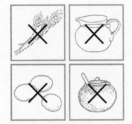

OVEN-BAKED CRAB CAKES

Makes 16 crab cakes (Serves 8)

Crab cakes are featured here as an appetizer, but you can make them larger for a main course. I like to keep Phillip's shelled and canned (pasteurized) crabmeat on hand so I can make crab cakes at a moment's notice.

1 pound shelled crabmeat
1 celery stalk, finely chopped
1 tablespoon dried minced onion,
   or 2 tablespoons grated fresh onion
2 teaspoons Seafood Seasoning
   (page 120)
1 tablespoon chopped fresh parsley
1 tablespoon Lea & Perrins
   Worcestershire sauce

1 teaspoon Italian seasoning
½ cup purchased mayonnaise
   or Homemade Mayonnaise
   (page 115)
1 tablespoon baking powder
1 cup gluten-free bread crumbs
Cocktail sauce, for dipping

1. Preheat oven to 400°F. Grease baking sheet or line with parchment paper.
2. Pick over shelled crabmeat. Combine all ingredients (except cocktail sauce) in food processor. Process until thoroughly mixed. Shape mixture into 16 small crab cakes. Arrange on prepared baking sheet.

3. Bake on lower rack for about 10 minutes per side, or until both sides are gently browned. Serve with cocktail sauce.

Nutrition Information (per serving)
Calories 110 • Fat 6g • Protein 7g • Carbohydrates 6g • Cholesterol 29mg • Sodium 443mg • Fiber .5g

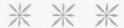

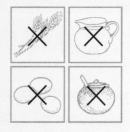

CHIP DIP

Makes 1½ cups (Serves 12)

This dip has much more flavor when made with the dairy ingredients. If dairy isn't appropriate for your diet, use the substitutes but you may need to boost the seasonings a bit. And a teaspoon of butter-flavored extract will help also.

1 package (8 ounces) cream cheese (cow or soy), at room temperature, or 1 package (10 ounces) soft silken tofu

4 ounces crumbled feta cheese, or ½ cup soft silken tofu

2 tablespoons 2% milk (cow, rice, or soy)

2 teaspoons Italian seasoning

1 to 2 garlic cloves (or to taste)

½ teaspoon cracked black pepper

Process all ingredients in food processor until very smooth. Add more milk, 1 tablespoon at a time, if mixture is too stiff. Garnish as desired. Serve with crackers, chips, or vegetables.

Nutrition Information (per 2-tablespoon serving)
Calories 80 • Fat 8g • Protein 2g • Carbohydrates 1g • Cholesterol 25mg • Sodium 110mg • Fiber 0.5g

Variation
Garnish with chopped green onion, black olives, tomatoes, chives, etc.

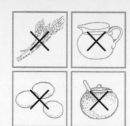

CHUTNEY APPETIZER SPREAD

Makes slightly less than 2 cups (Serves 6)

The sweet-and-spicy flavor of chutney melds wonderfully with creamy, mellow cream cheese (or tofu). This combination seems unlikely yet produces a wonderful taste sensation. And if you have the chutney on hand, you can whip this dish up in seconds. If you're not using cream cheese, add a teaspoon of butter-flavored extract to lend a "dairy" taste.

1 package (8 ounces) cream cheese (cow or soy), at room temperature, or 1 package (10 ounces) soft silken tofu

¼ cup chopped fresh cilantro, packed

2 tablespoons grated fresh onion

¼ teaspoon salt

¼ teaspoon white pepper

⅔ cup gluten-free mango chutney

¼ teaspoon crushed red pepper flakes

In food processor, process cream cheese, cilantro, onion, salt, and pepper. Stir in chutney and red pepper flakes. Refrigerate if not serving immediately.

Nutrition Information (per ⅓-cup serving)
Calories 166 • Fat 15g • Protein 3g • Carbohydrates 11g • Cholesterol 42mg • Sodium 415mg • Fiber 0.5g

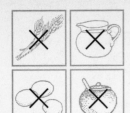

HOT SEAFOOD DIP

Makes about 2 cups (Serves 8)

If you don't use cream cheese yet want to replicate the dairy taste, try adding a teaspoon of butter-flavored extract.

1 cup cooked crabmeat

1 package (8 ounces) cream cheese (cow or soy), at room temperature, or 1 package (10 ounces) soft silken tofu

2 tablespoons Dijon mustard

1 tablespoon fresh lemon juice

1 teaspoon horseradish sauce, or ½ teaspoon fresh grated horseradish

2 tablespoons finely chopped onion

1 to 2 teaspoons Seafood Seasoning (page 120)

1 celery stalk, finely chopped

2 tablespoons fresh chopped parsley, for garnish

Dash paprika, for garnish

1. Prepare crabmeat by discarding any cartilage or bones. If crabmeat has been previously frozen or contains a lot of water, drain in a sieve while pressing firmly with a paper towel. Chop finely and set aside.
2. Combine cream cheese, mustard, lemon juice, horseradish sauce, onion, and seafood seasoning in food processor. Puree mixture until very smooth. Stir in celery and prepared crabmeat.
3. Spoon mixture into ovenproof bowl and heat to serving temperature, either by baking in a 350°F oven for 15–20 minutes or in microwave oven at Low-Medium setting until mixture reaches desired temperature.
4. Garnish with chopped parsley and dash of paprika. Serve hot with crackers or crispbread.

Nutrition Information (per ½-cup serving)
Calories 125 • Fat 11g • Protein 6g • Carbohydrates 2g • Cholesterol 46mg • Sodium 342mg • Fiber 5g

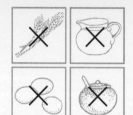

PRETZELS

Makes 30 pretzels

This recipe works best if you make the little stick-style pretzels.

1 tablespoon active dry yeast

½ cup sorghum flour or
brown rice flour

½ cup tapioca flour

2 teaspoons xanthan gum

½ teaspoon salt

1 teaspoon onion powder

1 teaspoon unflavored gelatin powder

⅔ cup warm 2% milk (cow, rice,
or soy) (110°F)

½ teaspoon sugar or honey

1 tablespoon olive oil

1 teaspoon vinegar

1 large egg white, beaten to foam*

1 tablespoon coarse salt (optional)

1. In medium mixer bowl, blend dry ingredients on low speed. Add milk, sugar, oil, and vinegar. Beat for 3 minutes at high speed. The batter will be soft.
2. Place dough in large, heavy-duty reclosable bag that has a ¼-inch opening cut diagonally on one corner. Squeeze dough through opening in straight sticks onto greased baking sheet. Hold bag upright to squeeze dough out. Also, hold bag with seam on top, rather than at side. Brush lightly with beaten egg white (or egg alternative). Place pretzels in warm place to rise 10–15 minutes, or until pretzels reach desired size.
3. Preheat oven to 400°F. Sprinkle pretzels with coarse salt (if using) and bake about 15 minutes, until they are dry and golden brown.

Nutrition Information (per pretzel)

Calories 30 • Fat 0.5g • Protein 1g • Carbohydrates 5g • Cholesterol 0mg • Sodium 228mg • Fiber 0.5g

*__Egg Alternative:__ Coat pretzels with cooking spray instead of egg wash.

Variation

For wider, softer pretzels cut opening ½ inch wide and remove pretzels from oven when lightly, not darkly, browned. (Optional: After first rising, immerse pretzels in 2 inches of simmering water with 1 tablespoon baking soda for 30 seconds, then return to baking sheet and bake as directed.) Store pretzels in airtight container to retain softness.

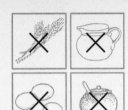

SAVORY CRACKERS

Makes about 20 crackers (Serves 10)

These crackers are very easy to make and also travel well. Try adding your favorite dried herbs for variety.

¼ cup sorghum flour or
   brown rice flour

¼ cup potato starch

¼ cup sweet rice flour

½ teaspoon xanthan gum

¼ teaspoon baking soda

½ teaspoon salt

2 tablespoons grated Parmesan cheese
   (cow, rice, or soy)

1 teaspoon onion powder,
   or 1 tablespoon grated fresh onion

2 tablespoons butter, melted, or
   canola oil

1 tablespoon honey or agave nectar

3 tablespoons toasted sesame seeds

2 tablespoons 2% milk (cow, rice,
   or soy)

1 teaspoon vinegar or fresh lemon juice

1. Preheat oven to 350°F. Grease baking sheet or line with parchment paper.
2. In food processor, combine flours, xanthan gum, baking soda, salt, Parmesan cheese, and onion powder. Add butter, honey, sesame seeds, milk, and vinegar. Mix until dough forms soft ball.
3. Shape dough into 20 balls, each 1 inch in diameter, and place on prepared baking sheet at least 2 inches apart. Using bottom of a drinking glass or rolling pin, flatten balls to approximately ⅛-inch thickness. Use fingers to smooth edges of the circle.
4. If you prefer not to hand-shape crackers, roll dough to ⅛-inch thickness on baking sheet. Then, using cookie cutter or biscuit cutter, cut crackers to desired shapes. Peel off unused dough and hand-shape these scraps into crackers.
5. Bake for 12–15 minutes, until crackers look firm and slightly toasted. Turn each cracker and bake another 5–7 minutes, or until golden brown. (Sprinkle with additional sesame seeds and salt, if desired.)

Nutrition Information (per serving)
Calories 50 • Fat 2g • Protein 1g • Carbohydrates 7g • Cholesterol 4mg • Sodium 91mg • Fiber 0.5g

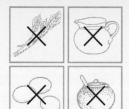

PARTY MIX

Makes 8 cups (Serves 16)

You can use any cereal you like in this dish as long as it's gluten-free. Remember that the larger the pieces are, the easier it will be to eat.

1 recipe Pretzels (page 85), or use Glutano brand pretzels

4 cups puffed corn, corn chips, or other cereal (Amaranth Snackers, see Resources, are a good choice.)

1 cup coarsely chopped pecans or walnuts

1 cup almonds or pumpkin seeds

½ cup sunflower seeds

¼ cup (½ stick) butter or margarine, melted, or use cooking spray

½ teaspoon garlic powder or onion powder

2 teaspoons Italian seasoning

1 tablespoon wheat-free tamari soy sauce

½ cup grated Parmesan cheese (cow, rice, or soy—may omit, but with some loss of flavor)

1 teaspoon paprika

1. Combine pretzels, cereal, nuts, and seeds in large bowl. Add melted butter to mixture, stirring until thoroughly coated. In small bowl, combine garlic powder, Italian seasoning, soy sauce, Parmesan cheese (if using), and paprika and stir until thoroughly mixed. Add to cereal mixture and toss until thoroughly coated. Spread mixture on large baking sheet.

2. Bake at 275°F for 45–50 minutes, or until mixture is lightly browned. Stir occasionally while mixture browns. Store in airtight container.

Nutrition Information (per ½-cup serving)
Calories 195 • Fat 15g • Protein 6g • Carbohydrates 10g • Cholesterol 10mg • Sodium 110mg • Fiber 3g

Variations

For a different taste sensation, replace soy sauce with gluten-free Worcestershire sauce and replace Italian seasoning with your favorite herb mix or gluten-free seasoned salt. You may use other cereals beside puffed corn, depending on your individual food sensitivities.

SALADS &
SALAD DRESSINGS

Salads are a marvelous way to add color, texture, and variety to your meals, and they are a source of important nutrients. A colorful, crunchy, flavorful salad adds pizzazz to any meal, but sometimes wheat, dairy, eggs, and cane sugar can show up in the form of croutons, salad dressings with wheat-flour thickener, and other unwanted surprises. You can enjoy the salads and salad dressings here without worry.

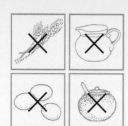

BALSAMIC VINEGAR DRESSING

Makes about ½ cup

Balsamic vinegar brings so much flavor to salads. You'll love this easy version.

>   2 tablespoons balsamic vinegar
>   1 tablespoon honey or agave nectar
>   Dash salt
>   ⅛ teaspoon xanthan gum
>   ¼ cup extra-virgin olive oil

Place balsamic vinegar, honey or agave nectar, salt, and xanthan gum in blender and process until blended. With blender on high, add oil in a steady stream and process until smooth. Refrigerate in airtight container.

Nutrition Information (per 1-tablespoon serving)
Calories 66 • Fat 7g • Protein 0g • Carbohydrates 2g • Cholesterol 0mg • Sodium 33mg • Fiber 0g

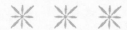

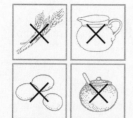

BASIC "VINAIGRETTE"

Makes about ½ cup

This basic "vinaigrette" doesn't have vinegar, so it's a bit less acidic.

>   ¼ cup Chicken Stock (page 110)
>   1 tablespoon extra-virgin olive oil
>   2 teaspoons Dijon mustard
>
>   1 garlic clove, minced
>   ¼ teaspoon salt
>   ⅛ teaspoon black pepper

In small bowl, whisk together ingredients until thoroughly mixed. Or process in a blender or small food processor. Refrigerate in airtight container. Shake just before serving.

Nutrition Information (per 2-tablespoon serving)
Calories 35 • Fat 4g • Protein 1g • Carbohydrates 1g • Cholesterol 0mg • Sodium 400mg • Fiber 1g

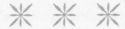

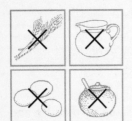

CITRUS DRESSING

Makes about ½ cup

I like to serve this dressing on salads where fish or poultry is featured on the menu.

2 tablespoons fresh lemon juice

¼ cup fresh orange juice

2 teaspoons fresh lime juice

2 tablespoons olive oil

1 tablespoon grated orange zest

2 teaspoons grated lime zest

2 teaspoons dried basil leaves

2 teaspoons fennel seeds

¼ teaspoon crushed red pepper flakes

⅛ teaspoon salt

⅛ teaspoon xanthan gum

Dash white pepper

Combine all ingredients in blender and process until well blended. Refrigerate in airtight container for up to 1 week.

Nutrition Information (per 1-tablespoon serving)
Calories 35 • Fat 4g • Protein 0g • Carbohydrates 1g • Cholesterol 0mg • Sodium 90mg • Fiber 0g

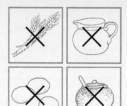

FRENCH DRESSING

Makes about ¾ cup

French dressing is the classic dressing for so many salads.

2 tablespoons vinegar

2 tablespoons fresh lemon juice

2 teaspoons granulated sugar or
fructose powder

½ teaspoon salt

½ teaspoon dry mustard

½ teaspoon paprika

¼ teaspoon white pepper

⅛ teaspoon xanthan gum

Dash cayenne pepper

2 tablespoons water

⅓ cup canola oil

Place all ingredients, except oil, in blender and process until smooth. With motor running, add oil and process until smooth. Refrigerate in airtight container. Shake just before serving.

Nutrition Information (per 2-tablespoon serving)
Calories 60 • Fat 6g • Protein 0g • Carbohydrates 1g • Cholesterol 0mg • Sodium 90mg • Fiber 0g

Note: You can make your own dry mustard by grinding mustard seeds in a small coffee grinder.

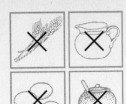

ITALIAN DRESSING

Makes 1½ cups

This dressing may have a lot of ingredients, but the end result is fantastic.

½ cup cider vinegar

¼ teaspoon dried oregano leaves

½ teaspoon freeze-dried chives

½ teaspoon dried parsley flakes

¼ teaspoon dry mustard

⅛ teaspoon white pepper

⅛ teaspoon garlic powder or fresh garlic, minced

½ teaspoon salt

½ teaspoon grated Parmesan cheese (cow, rice, or soy)

1 tablespoon chopped onion

½ teaspoon honey or agave nectar

⅛ teaspoon xanthan gum

Dash cayenne pepper

½ cup extra-virgin olive oil

½ cup water or gluten-free chicken broth

Process all ingredients in blender. Refrigerate in airtight container.

Nutrition Information (per 1-tablespoon serving)
Calories 40 • Fat 5g • Protein 0g • Carbohydrates 1g • Cholesterol 0mg • Sodium 45mg • Fiber 0.5g

Note: You can make your own dry mustard by grinding mustard seeds in a small coffee grinder.

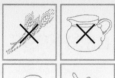
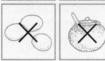

LEMON "VINAIGRETTE"

Makes 1 cup

Although this wonderfully fresh "vinaigrette" is great on salads, I also like to use it on grilled fish.

½ cup fresh lemon juice

2 tablespoons olive oil

1 tablespoon honey or agave nectar

1 garlic clove, minced

1 tablespoon Dijon mustard

1 teaspoon dried oregano

1 teaspoon dried parsley

½ teaspoon crushed fennel seeds

½ teaspoon salt

⅛ teaspoon crushed red pepper flakes

⅛ teaspoon xanthan gum

Dash white pepper

Process all ingredients in blender until smooth. Refrigerate in airtight container. Shake well before serving.

Nutrition Information (per 1-tablespoon serving)
Calories 20 • Fat 2g • Protein 1g • Carbohydrates 2g • Cholesterol 0mg • Sodium 80mg • Fiber 0.5g

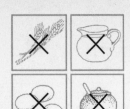

LIME-CILANTRO DRESSING

Makes about 1 cup

The lime in this dressing provides a pleasing alternative to the usual lemon dressing and complements meals with a Southwestern theme.

½ cup extra-virgin olive oil

¼ cup water

¼ cup fresh lime juice

¼ cup fresh lemon juice

¼ cup chopped fresh cilantro

1 teaspoon grated lime zest

½ teaspoon salt

1 medium garlic clove, minced

½ teaspoon honey or agave
   nectar

⅛ teaspoon ground cumin

⅛ teaspoon xanthan gum

Process all ingredients in blender until smooth. Refrigerate in airtight container for up to 1 week.

Nutrition Information (per 1-tablespoon serving)

Calories 65 • Fat 7g • Protein 0g • Carbohydrates 1g • Cholesterol 0mg • Sodium 65mg • Fiber 0.5g

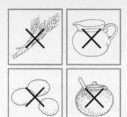

ORIENTAL DRESSING

Makes about 1 cup

Try this dressing on an Oriental tossed salad or on rice or pure buckwheat noodles.

½ cup rice vinegar
¼ cup olive oil
2 tablespoons fresh lemon juice
1 garlic clove, minced
2 tablespoons light brown sugar
   or maple sugar

1 teaspoon dried mint, or 6 fresh
   mint leaves
2 thin slices peeled fresh gingerroot
⅛ teaspoon xanthan gum
Dash cayenne pepper
Dash salt and pepper

Process all ingredients in blender until smooth. Store in airtight container in refrigerator.

Nutrition Information (per 1-tablespoon serving)
Calories 45 • Fat 4g • Protein 1g • Carbohydrates 50g • Cholesterol 0mg • Sodium 2mg •
   Fiber 0.5g

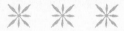

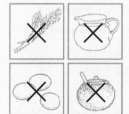

RANCH DRESSING

Makes 1 cup

This homey dressing is great on salads or drizzled over baked potatoes.

½ cup purchased mayonnaise
   or Homemade Mayonnaise
   (page 115)

½ cup 2% milk (cow, rice, or soy)
¼ teaspoon onion salt
⅛ teaspoon garlic salt

¼ teaspoon black pepper

¼ teaspoon dried marjoram leaves

¼ teaspoon celery salt

¼ teaspoon dried savory leaves

¼ teaspoon dried parsley

Process all ingredients in blender until smooth. Refrigerate in airtight container for up to 1 week.

Nutrition Information (per 1-tablespoon serving)
Calories 55 • Fat 5g • Protein 1g • Carbohydrates 1g • Cholesterol 5mg • Sodium 56mg • Fiber 0g

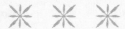

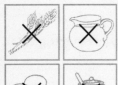

SESAME DRESSING

Makes 1 cup

Choose this dressing to add flavor to any Asian dish.

½ cup rice vinegar

¼ cup canola oil

¼ cup sesame oil

2 teaspoons salt

2 teaspoons honey or agave nectar

2 tablespoons grated orange zest

1 small garlic clove, minced

1 teaspoon ground black pepper

1 teaspoon peeled fresh gingerroot

1 teaspoon wheat-free tamari soy sauce

¼ teaspoon crushed red pepper flakes

⅛ teaspoon xanthan gum

Process all ingredients in blender until smooth. Refrigerate in airtight container. Shake before serving.

Nutrition Information (per 1-tablespoon serving)
Calories 65 • Fat 7g • Protein 1g • Carbohydrates 2g • Cholesterol 0mg • Sodium 285mg • Fiber 0.5g

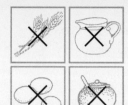

SOY DRESSING

Makes about ½ cup

This slightly spicy dressing is great on Asian dishes.

2 tablespoons wheat-free tamari
   soy sauce
2 tablespoons canola oil
1 tablespoon rice vinegar
1 tablespoon chopped fresh cilantro
   (optional)
1 serrano chile, seeded and chopped*

1 teaspoon sesame oil
1 teaspoon honey or agave nectar
¼ teaspoon salt
¼ teaspoon black pepper
⅛ teaspoon xanthan gum
Juice of 1 lime

Process all ingredients in blender until smooth. Refrigerate in airtight container.

Nutrition Information (per 1-tablespoon serving)
Calories 45 • Fat 4g • Protein 1g • Carbohydrates 2g • Cholesterol 0mg • Sodium 275mg •
   Fiber 0.5g

*Wear gloves while cutting serrano chile.

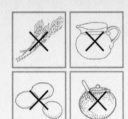

THOUSAND ISLAND DRESSING

Makes 1¼ cups

This classic dressing is great on salads and is also the sauce commonly used in Reuben sandwiches.

1 cup purchased mayonnaise
   or Homemade Mayonnaise
   (page 115)

3 tablespoons Chili Sauce (page 99)

1 tablespoon chopped green bell
   pepper

1 teaspoon chopped canned pimientos
   (optional)

1 teaspoon dried chives,
   or 1 tablespoon chopped
   fresh chives

Process all ingredients in blender until smooth. Refrigerate in airtight container.

Nutrition Information (per 1-tablespoon serving)
Calories 80 • Fat 9g • Protein 0g • Carbohydrates 1g • Cholesterol 6mg • Sodium 65mg • Fiber 0g

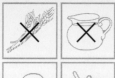

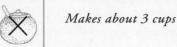

CHILI SAUCE

Makes about 3 cups

Use this tasty sauce on meat and as an ingredient in Thousand Island Dressing (page 98).

6 large tomatoes, peeled and chopped
2 large onions, finely chopped
2 green bell peppers, finely chopped
¾ cup granulated sugar or fructose powder
½ cup vinegar
1 teaspoon celery seeds

¾ teaspoon salt
¼ teaspoon ground cinnamon
¼ teaspoon ground cloves
¼ teaspoon ground ginger
¼ teaspoon crushed red pepper flakes
¼ teaspoon dry mustard

Combine all ingredients in large saucepan over low-medium heat. Simmer gently for 45–60 minutes, uncovered, until thickened. Stir frequently to prevent sticking. Remove from heat and cool slightly. Refrigerate in airtight container.

Nutrition Information (per 2-tablespoon serving)
Calories 35 • Fat 0.5g • Protein 1g • Carbohydrates 8g • Cholesterol 0mg • Sodium 115mg • Fiber 0.5g

Note: You can make your own dry mustard by grinding mustard seeds in a small coffee grinder.

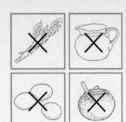

TOMATO-BASIL VINAIGRETTE

Makes about ½ cup

This dressing is especially nice in the summer when tomatoes are in season.

2 large tomatoes, seeded and chopped

2 tablespoons red wine vinegar or fresh lemon or lime juice

2 tablespoons extra-virgin olive oil

1 tablespoon dried basil leaves

½ teaspoon dried oregano leaves

½ teaspoon garlic powder, or 1 garlic clove, minced

½ teaspoon sugar or honey

¼ teaspoon salt

¼ teaspoon black pepper

Process all ingredients in blender until smooth. Refrigerate in airtight container for up to 2 days.

Nutrition Information (per 2-tablespoon serving)
Calories 85 • Fat 7g • Protein 1g • Carbohydrates 6g • Cholesterol 0mg • Sodium 152mg • Fiber 1g

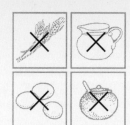

VINEGAR~FREE
HERB DRESSING

Makes about ¾ cup

My favorite herbs are thyme, basil, marjoram, and savory—but use the ones you like.

½ cup fresh lemon juice

¼ extra-virgin olive oil

2 small garlic cloves

2 teaspoons honey or agave nectar

½ cup chopped green onions or chives

3 teaspoons dried herbs of choice

½ teaspoon salt

⅛ teaspoon xanthan gum
  (optional)

⅛ teaspoon black pepper

Process all ingredients in blender until smooth. Best when served immediately.

Nutrition Information (per 2-tablespoon serving)
Calories 100 • Fat 9g • Protein 0g • Carbohydrates 5g • Cholesterol 0mg • Sodium 195mg •
  Fiber 1g

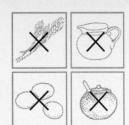

CAESAR SALAD WITHOUT EGGS

Serves 4

Use only half of the garlic-oil mixture to toss with the croutons, adding the remainder to the salad dressing itself. Although the traditional version of this salad is made with eggs, you won't even miss them.

2 garlic cloves

¼ cup extra-virgin olive oil

½ teaspoon salt

1 cup gluten-free croutons

1 tablespoon fresh lemon juice

1 teaspoon vinegar or fresh lemon juice

1 teaspoon dry mustard

1 teaspoon Lea & Perrins Worcestershire sauce

1 teaspoon anchovy paste (Reese) (optional)

1 head Romaine lettuce, washed and torn

⅓ cup grated Parmesan cheese (cow, rice, or soy)

1. Use garlic press to mince garlic before mashing with olive oil and salt. Brown croutons for 10 minutes in a 350°F oven. Toss with half of garlic-oil mixture and return to oven for another 3–5 minutes, until golden. Remove from oven and set aside until cool.

2. In large salad bowl, whisk together remaining garlic-oil mixture, lemon juice, vinegar, mustard, Worcestershire sauce, and anchovy paste (if using). Add Romaine lettuce and toss thoroughly. Sprinkle with Parmesan cheese and croutons, toss again, and serve immediately.

Nutrition Information (per serving)
Calories 210 • Fat 17g • Protein 6g • Carbohydrates 10g • Cholesterol 5mg • Sodium 467mg • Fiber 4g

Note: You can make your own dry mustard by grinding mustard seeds in a small coffee grinder.

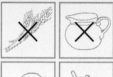

POTATO SALAD

Makes about 5 cups (Serves 6)

If eggs are not appropriate for your diet, omit them and use another potato instead to make the salad egg free.

3 cups peeled and diced cooked potatoes
4 hard-cooked eggs, peeled and chopped
½ cup finely chopped celery
¼ cup finely chopped green onion
2 tablespoons sweet pickle relish, or 2 teaspoons dried dill weed

½ cup Homemade Mayonnaise (page 115)
1 tablespoon vinegar
1 teaspoon sugar or honey
½ teaspoon celery salt
½ teaspoon celery seeds
¼ teaspoon white pepper
½ teaspoon dry mustard
Paprika, for garnish

Combine potatoes, eggs, celery, onion, and relish in large bowl. In small bowl, whisk all remaining ingredients except paprika until smooth. Pour over potato mixture and toss until thoroughly coated. Turn into serving bowl and sprinkle with paprika. Refrigerate until serving time.

Nutrition Information (per serving)
Calories 165 • Fat 7g • Protein 6g • Carbohydrates 19g • Cholesterol 146mg • Sodium 280mg • Fiber 2g

Note: You can make your own dry mustard by grinding mustard seeds in a small coffee grinder.

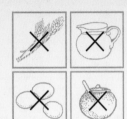

SPINACH SALAD WITH STRAWBERRIES

Serves 10

Try mixing in a few green or red grapes for added interest.

3 tablespoons fresh orange juice

1 tablespoon fresh lemon juice

1 tablespoon honey or agave nectar

2 tablespoons dried basil leaves

¼ teaspoon dried thyme leaves

¼ teaspoon xanthan gum

⅛ teaspoon cayenne pepper

⅛ teaspoon salt

⅛ teaspoon white pepper

¼ cup olive oil or canola oil

1 package (10 ounces) baby spinach leaves, rinsed and dried

1 pint hulled strawberries, rinsed and dried

1 cup pecan halves, toasted

¼ cup crumbled feta cheese (omit if you are dairy sensitive)

1. In small jar, whisk together orange juice, lemon juice, honey or agave nectar, basil, thyme, xanthan gum, cayenne pepper, salt, white pepper, and oil until smooth.
2. Place cleaned spinach leaves in large bowl. Halve strawberries and add along with pecans. Add enough dressing to coat leaves and toss gently. Just before serving, sprinkle crumbled feta cheese on top.

Nutrition Information (per serving)
Calories 160 • Fat 15g • Protein 2g • Carbohydrates 7g • Cholesterol 3mg • Sodium 71mg • Fiber 2g

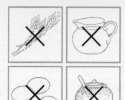

WALDORF SALAD

Serves 4

We have this salad often at my house to make sure we're getting enough fruits and vegetables plus lots of fiber in our diet.

2 Red Delicious apples, cut into
    ½-inch cubes
2 celery stalks, chopped into
    ¾-inch cubes
½ cup pecan halves, toasted
½ cup golden raisins

1 teaspoon fresh lemon juice
2 tablespoons Homemade
    Mayonnaise (page 115)
⅛ teaspoon salt
½ teaspoon granulated sugar or
    fructose powder

Combine apples, celery, pecans, and raisins in small bowl. In another bowl, stir together lemon juice, mayonnaise, salt, and sugar or fructose powder. Pour mayonnaise mixture over apple mixture and toss thoroughly. Serve immediately.

Nutrition Information (per serving)
Calories 225 • Fat 12g • Protein 2g • Carbohydrates 32g • Cholesterol 2mg • Sodium 130mg •
    Fiber 4g

INGREDIENTS &
CONDIMENTS

S ometimes it's the simple, little ingredients that
cause the most difficulty for people on special
diets. This section contains recipes for condiments and simple baking ingredients we never think about
until our special diets force us to re-examine everything
that goes in our mouth.

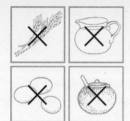

BAKING POWDER
WITH CORN

Makes about ½ cup (or 24 teaspoons)

If you can't eat corn, try the grain-free version (see next recipe).

> ¼ cup cream of tartar
> 3 tablespoons cornstarch
> 2 tablespoons baking soda

Mix cream of tartar, cornstarch, and baking soda together in glass jar and store in cool, dark place for up to 1 month. Use in same proportions as baking powder.

Nutrition Information (per 1-teaspoon serving)
Calories 8 • Fat 0g • Protein 0g • Carbohydrates 2g • Cholesterol 0mg • Sodium 316mg • Fiber 0g

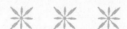

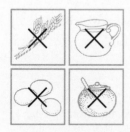

BAKING POWDER
WITHOUT CORN

Makes ¾ cup (or 36 teaspoons)

When a recipe calls for 1 teaspoon baking powder, you may use 1½ teaspoons of this corn-free version. Make this frequently rather than doubling it—it loses potency over time.

> ⅓ cup cream of tartar
> ⅓ cup arrowroot
> 3 tablespoons baking soda

Mix cream of tartar, arrowroot, and baking soda together in glass jar and store in cool, dark place for up to 1 month.

Nutrition Information (per 1-teaspoon serving)
Calories 8 • Fat 0g • Protein 0g • Carbohydrates 2g • Cholesterol 0mg • Sodium 315mg • Fiber 0g

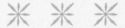

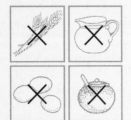

FLAX (FLAXSEED) MIX

Makes 1 cup

This egg substitute works best in recipes with a darker color where you are replacing one egg rather than two. It works best as a binder and moisturizer, but it is not a leavening agent as are eggs. Therefore, baked goods will be heavier and denser.

3 teaspoons flaxseed or flaxseed meal
1 cup boiling water

Grind seeds into a fine powder in a coffee grinder or use flaxseed meal which is already ground. Whisk into boiling water, remove from heat, and let stand for 5 minutes. Use as a substitute for eggs—¼ cup flax mix equals 1 large egg.

Nutrition Information (per ¼ cup)
Calories 15 • Fat 1g • Protein <1g • Carbohydrates 1g • Cholesterol 0mg • Sodium 3mg • Fiber 1g

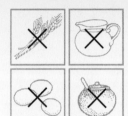

BEEF STOCK

Makes about 4 quarts

This version produces a deeper, more fully flavored beef stock because the beef and vegetables are roasted. If you don't have time to roast the ingredients—or prefer a milder stock—simply simmer the ingredients together for a couple of hours. I prefer to use an ovenproof Dutch oven that goes from oven to stove top, thus eliminating an extra pan. See the recipes for Chicken Stock and Vegetable Stock on pages 110 and 111.

1 pound beef stew meat, cut into 1-inch cubes	1 bunch parsley
1 large onion, peeled and quartered	1 teaspoon dried thyme leaves
1 large carrot, sliced lengthwise	¼ teaspoon dill seed
1 large celery stalk, halved	1 teaspoon salt
2 large garlic cloves, peeled	6 whole black peppercorns
4 quarts cold water	1 large bay leaf
	1 large tomato, halved

1. Place the beef, onion, and carrot in large greased roasting pan and roast for 20–30 minutes in a 400°F oven until nicely browned. Transfer vegetables to large stockpot and add remaining ingredients. Pour off any extra fat from roasting pan and add just enough water to cover bottom of pan. Deglaze pan over medium-high heat, scraping up browned bits. Add this mixture to stockpot.

2. Bring mixture in stockpot slowly to a simmer, cover, and continue to simmer for 3 hours. (Avoid bringing to boil rapidly, since this produces foam that you'll have to skim off.)

3. Strain stock through a sieve. Chill stock and remove any fat that rises to top. If you're not using all stock immediately, freeze it for up to 3 months.

Nutrition Information (per 1-cup serving)
Calories 8 • Fat 1g • Protein 0g • Carbohydrates 2g • Cholesterol 0mg • Sodium 156mg • Fiber 1g

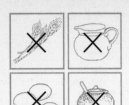

CHICKEN STOCK

Makes 3 quarts

Save the bones from Sunday's roast chicken and use them to flavor this stock. If you refrigerate the stock, the fat can easily be skimmed off the following day and frozen in containers. For Beef Stock recipe, see page 109. For Vegetable Stock recipe, see page 111.

3 quarts water

2 pounds chicken pieces or bones

1 tablespoon salt

1 small onion, halved

4 celery stalks, leaves left on

4 large carrots, peeled

2 small parsnips (optional)

6 dill seeds

6 whole black peppercorns

1 large tomato, halved

1 bunch fresh herbs (thyme, savory, marjoram, etc.), or 2 teaspoons dried herbs of choice

Combine all ingredients in large stockpot. Bring to a simmer slowly, cover tightly, and let cook for 2–3 hours. Let stock cool in refrigerator. Skim off any fat. Strain stock through a fine mesh sieve and discard solids. Freeze in tightly covered containers.

Nutrition Information (per 1-cup serving)
Calories 40 • Fat 0.5g • Protein 1g • Carbohydrates 9g • Cholesterol 0mg • Sodium 670mg • Fiber 2g

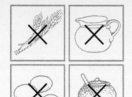

VEGETABLE STOCK

Makes 3 quarts (Serves 12)

Keep jars of this flavorful stock in your freezer and you'll always be prepared.

3 quarts water
1 tablespoon salt
1 small onion, halved
4 celery stalks, leaves left on
4 large carrots, peeled
2 small parsnips (optional)

6 dill seeds
6 whole black peppercorns
1 large tomato, halved
1 bunch fresh herbs (thyme,
   marjoram, savory, etc.), or
2 teaspoons dried herbs of choice

Combine all ingredients in large stockpot. Bring to simmer slowly, cover tightly, and cook for 2–3 hours. Let stock cool in refrigerator. Strain stock through fine mesh sieve and discard solids. Freeze in tightly covered containers.

Nutrition Information (per 1-cup serving)
Calories 40 • Fat 0g • Protein 0g • Carbohydrates 9g • Cholesterol 0mg • Sodium 670mg • Fiber 2g

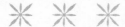

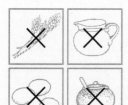

ITALIAN BREAD CRUMBS

Makes 2 cups

Italian bread crumbs are so easy to make and add so much flavor to our gluten-free diet. If you prefer them dry, toast them in a slow oven to desired degree of dryness.

4 cups gluten-free bread, torn into small pieces
4 teaspoons Italian seasoning
1 teaspoon onion powder

Place bread in food processor and pulse on/off until crumbs reach desired consistency. Toss with remaining ingredients. Store tightly covered, in refrigerator, for up to 2 weeks.

Nutrition Information (per 1-tablespoon serving)
Calories 65 • Fat 1g • Protein 2g • Carbohydrates 12g • Cholesterol 1mg • Sodium 114mg • Fiber 1g

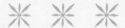

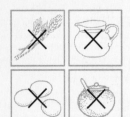

NUT MILK

Makes about 2 cups

The nice thing about making your own nut milk is that you can vary the ingredients to achieve the desired result. For example, for a sweeter version simply increase the sweetener. Likewise, for a less sweet version to be used for savory dishes, omit the sweetener altogether. Vary the density of the milk by increasing the nuts and/or decreasing the amount of water.

> ½ cup raw cashews or almonds
> 2 cups water
> 1 teaspoon honey or agave nectar
> ½ teaspoon vanilla extract (optional)

Combine ingredients in blender and process about 5 minutes, until completely smooth. Strain through cheesecloth to remove any remaining nuts. Refrigerate, covered, for up to 1 week. Use in dishes as you would use any nondairy milk substitute.

Nutrition Information (per ½-cup serving)
Calories 105 • Fat 8g • Protein 3g • Carbohydrates 7g • Cholesterol 0mg • Sodium 6mg • Fiber 1g

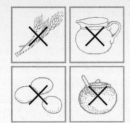

RICE MILK

Makes about 3 cups

The advantage to making your own rice milk is that you can vary the density of the milk by increasing the rice and/or decreasing the amount of water. The cashews add flavor and body, but they can be omitted. I prefer using basmati rice, but you can also use plain white or brown rice.

3 cups warm water	1 tablespoon honey or agave
⅔ cup hot cooked rice	nectar (or to taste)
⅓ cup raw cashews	1 teaspoon vanilla extract
(optional)	⅛ teaspoon xanthan gum

Process all ingredients in blender until very, very smooth. Strain through cheesecloth to remove any remaining rice particles. Refrigerate, covered, for up to 1 week.

Nutrition Information (per ¼-cup serving)
Calories 25 • Fat 0g • Protein 0g • Carbohydrates 5g • Cholesterol 0mg • Sodium 3mg • Fiber 0g

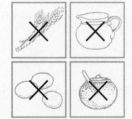

SOUR "CREAM"

Makes 1½ cups (Serves 20)

Use this easy sour cream any way you would use regular sour cream. It may not be quite as white as the dairy-based sour cream you're accustomed to using.

1 package (10.5–12 ounces) soft silken tofu
2 tablespoons vinegar or fresh lemon juice
1 tablespoon fresh lemon juice
1 teaspoon butter extract

Process all ingredients in food processor until very smooth. Refrigerate in airtight container.

Nutrition Information (per serving)
Calories 10 • Fat 0.5g • Protein 1g • Carbohydrates 1g • Cholesterol 0mg • Sodium 6mg • Fiber 0g

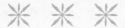

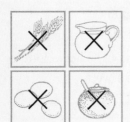

YOGURT CHEESE

Makes 14 tablespoons (⅞ cup)

This is a great way to get a cream-cheese-like product without the fat. The rice or soy version may not drain as thoroughly as the cow's-milk version.

8 ounces plain nonfat yogurt (cow, rice, or soy)

Place yogurt in strainer lined with cheesecloth or paper coffee filter. Refrigerate, covered, for 24 hours. Discard liquid. Refrigerate for up to 1 week.

Nutrition Information (per serving)
Calories 10 • Fat 0g • Protein 1g • Carbohydrates 1g • Cholesterol 0mg • Sodium 11mg • Fiber 0g

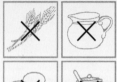
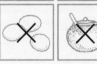

HOMEMADE MAYONNAISE

Makes about 1 cup

After you make this easy mayonnaise recipe once, you may alter the ingredients to achieve your preferred taste. Here, it's really more like a tangy salad dressing. For a less tangy version, reduce the vinegar or increase the sugar for a sweeter spread. Use this mayonnaise the same way you would use commercial mayonnaise. It tastes so good, it's hard to believe it has no dairy or eggs.

¼ cup canola oil or safflower oil
¼ cup water
2 tablespoons fresh lemon juice
2 tablespoons vinegar or Ener-G yeast-free vinegar powder, reconstituted
2 teaspoons sweet-rice flour
1 teaspoon arrowroot

½ teaspoon xanthan gum
½ teaspoon granulated sugar or fructose powder
¼ teaspoon dry mustard
¼ teaspoon salt
⅛ teaspoon white pepper
⅛ teaspoon cayenne pepper

Combine all ingredients in blender and process until mixture thickens. Store in refrigerator for up to 1 week.

Nutrition Information (per 2-tablespoon serving)
Calories 65 • Fat 7g • Protein 0g • Carbohydrates 2g • Cholesterol 0mg • Sodium 72mg • Fiber 0g

Note: You can make your own dry mustard by grinding mustard seeds in a small coffee grinder.

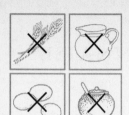

MUSTARD

Makes 1 cup

It's not hard to make your own mustard, and once you get the hang of it you can experiment with different flavors, too.

3 tablespoons tapioca flour

⅔ cup water, divided

¼ cup dry mustard

⅓ cup vinegar

2 tablespoons honey

½ teaspoon salt

2 tablespoons fresh grated
   horseradish

¼ teaspoon ground turmeric

⅛ teaspoon paprika

1. Mix tapioca flour in ¼ cup of the water to form a paste and set aside.
2. In small saucepan over low-medium heat, mix together dry mustard, vinegar, honey, salt, and remainder of water. Gradually whisk in tapioca-flour paste until well blended. Bring to boil, stirring constantly, until mixture thickens.
3. Remove from heat and stir in horseradish, turmeric, and paprika. Refrigerate in airtight container for up to 1 week.

Nutrition Information (per 2-tablespoon serving)
Calories 30 • Fat 0g • Protein 0g • Carbohydrates 8g • Cholesterol 0mg • Sodium 145mg •
   Fiber 0g

Note: You can make your own dry mustard by grinding mustard seeds in a small coffee grinder.

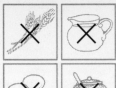
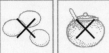

TOMATO KETCHUP

Makes 4 cups

Adjust the spices to suit your family's tastes. You may halve the recipe, if you wish.

1 can (35 ounces) tomatoes
¼ cup vinegar
¼ cup packed light brown sugar
2 garlic cloves, minced
2 tablespoons peeled, grated fresh
   gingerroot
1 teaspoon ground cumin

¼ teaspoon cayenne pepper
½ teaspoon ground cinnamon
½ teaspoon salt
¼ teaspoon black pepper
⅛ teaspoon ground allspice
⅛ teaspoon ground cloves

1. Place all ingredients in medium, heavy saucepan and bring to boil. Reduce to low and simmer, uncovered, for 1 hour, or until liquid evaporates. Stir occasionally to avoid scorching. Let cool for 15 minutes.
2. Transfer mixture to food processor and puree until very smooth. Refrigerate, covered, for up to 2 weeks.

Nutrition Information (per 2-tablespoon serving)
Calories 10 • Fat 0g • Protein 0g • Carbohydrates 3g • Cholesterol 0mg • Sodium 39 mg •
   Fiber 0.5g

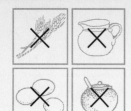

BREADING MIX

Makes 2 cups (or 32 tablespoons)

This easy breading mix is extremely versatile. You can use it for meats, seafood, or vegetables when frying.

1 cup potato flour (not potato starch)	1 teaspoon baking powder
1 cup arrowroot	1 teaspoon salt
1 teaspoon dried thyme leaves	½ teaspoon cayenne pepper
1 teaspoon dried oregano leaves	¼ teaspoon garlic powder
1 teaspoon onion powder	¼ teaspoon sugar

Mix ingredients together and store in airtight container in dark, dry place. Use as breading mix for meats, seafood, or vegetables in frying and baking. Do not reuse the mix after dipping raw food into it. Use within 3 months.

Nutrition Information (per 1-tablespoon serving)
Calories 35 • Fat 6g • Protein .5g • Carbohydrates 8g • Cholesterol 0mg • Sodium 80mg • Fiber .5g

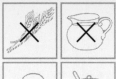

ONION SOUP MIX

Makes about ⅔ cup (about 11 tablespoons)

This tasty onion soup mix is great for making chip dips, gravy, or for sprinkling on beef roasts.

½ cup dried minced onions
1 teaspoon onion salt
1 tablespoon sweet-rice flour
½ teaspoon boullion granules*

¼ teaspoon garlic powder
¼ teaspoon granulated sugar or
  fructose powder
¼ teaspoon apple pectin powder

Shake ingredients in screw-top jar to blend. Store mixture in dark, dry place. Use in the same proportions as commercial onion soup mix. Double or triple recipe, if needed.

Nutrition Information (per 1-tablespoon serving)
Calories 15 • Fat 0g • Protein .5g • Carbohydrates 3g • Cholesterol 0mg • Sodium 160mg • Fiber .5g

*Ener-G brand is gluten-free.

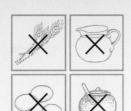

SEAFOOD SEASONING

Makes about 6 tablespoons

Use this seasoning on your favorite seafood by rubbing it on all sides of the fish and then refrigerate for at least 1 hour. Cook as directed.

1 tablespoon dried thyme leaves

1 tablespoon dried sage leaves

1 tablespoon dried marjoram leaves

1 tablespoon dried savory leaves

2 teaspoons freeze-dried chives

1 small bay leaf, crushed

1 teaspoon paprika

1 teaspoon celery salt

½ teaspoon mustard powder

½ teaspoon onion powder

¼ teaspoon ground ginger

¼ teaspoon ground nutmeg

¼ teaspoon ground cardamom

¼ teaspoon cayenne pepper

⅛ teaspoon ground cloves

Combine all ingredients in glass jar with tight-fitting lid. Store in a dark, cool place up to 3 months.

Nutrition Information (per 1-tablespoon serving)
Calories 11 • Fat 0g • Protein .5g • Carbohydrates 2g • Cholesterol 0mg • Sodium 265mg • Fiber .5g

MAIN DISHES

Whether you're fixing a quick weeknight meal for your family or a more leisurely weekend dinner, you'll find plenty of flavorful dishes in this chapter that will please anyone who can't eat wheat, dairy, eggs, or cane sugar.

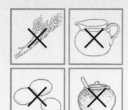

BARBECUED CHICKEN

Serves 4

This sauce is so simple and easy. You can make it the day before and chill, and it is ready to use when you need it.

1 can (5.5 ounces) tomato juice
¼ cup fresh lemon juice
1 tablespoon butter or margarine
1 teaspoon grated lemon zest
1 teaspoon Lea & Perrins
  Worcestershire sauce

½ teaspoon onion powder
¼ teaspoon black pepper
¼ teaspoon cayenne pepper
1 garlic clove, minced
1 pound chicken legs and thighs

Combine all ingredients except chicken in small, heavy saucepan. Simmer over low-medium heat for 10–15 minutes. Brush sauce on chicken as it grills.

Nutrition Information (per serving)
Calories 190 • Fat 9g • Protein 24g • Carbohydrates 4g • Cholesterol 80mg • Sodium 225mg • Fiber 0.5g

BACKYARD BARBECUE

Barbecued Chicken (page 122)

Potato Salad (page 103)

Garlic French Bread (page 16)

Chocolate Ice-Cream Sandwiches (page 229)

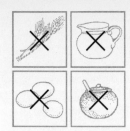

CORNISH GAME HENS WITH FRUIT GLAZE

Serves 4

These are especially pretty to serve on a large platter surrounded by your favorite cooked rice. The fruit glaze provides a wonderful complement to the crispy skin and assures a beautifully browned bird.

2 Cornish game hens, halved	1 teaspoon olive oil
½ teaspoon salt	¼ teaspoon dried thyme leaves
¼ teaspoon black pepper	¼ teaspoon dried tarragon leaves
½ cup raspberry jam	1 small garlic clove, minced
¼ cup red wine vinegar	

1. Wash game hens and pat dry. Season with salt and pepper. Arrange game hens skin side up in oiled roasting pan. If possible, place hens on roasting rack in pan so they do not sit in fat while roasting.
2. Combine remaining ingredients in small bowl to make glaze and microwave until jam is melted. Stir mixture thoroughly.
3. Bake hens, covered, in a 400°F oven for 45–60 minutes, brushing frequently with glaze.

Nutrition Information (per serving)
Calories 400 • Fat 25g • Protein 29g • Carbohydrates 12g • Cholesterol 170mg • Sodium 400mg • Fiber 1g

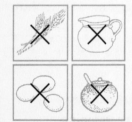

TURKEY WITH GRAVY

This recipe works best with a fresh turkey (which has no questionable additives). The brining imparts moisture and flavor and works best with a turkey under 14 pounds because it will fit into a large pot.

1 cup coarse or kosher salt	½ teaspoon ground allspice
⅓ cup honey	6 black peppercorns, crushed
2 large bay leaves	2 gallons water, divided
1 tablespoon dried thyme leaves	1 fresh turkey, 14 pounds or less
6 whole cloves	Gravy (page 125)

1. In very large stockpot or canning pot, combine salt, honey, bay leaves, thyme, cloves, allspice, peppercorns, and 2 cups water. Bring to boil, stirring until salt dissolves. Remove from heat and add remaining water. Let cool.
2. Rinse fresh turkey; check for pinfeathers. Remove giblets; wash cavities thoroughly. Place turkey breast side down in brine, covering completely. If not, add more water. Cover and refrigerate overnight.
3. Rinse turkey; discard brine.
4. Pat turkey dry. Do not add additional salt. Place in large roaster pan and roast at 350°F, basting frequently. Turkey is done when a thermometer inserted into breast meat registers 180°F. Remove turkey from oven and let sit in roasting pan, covered, 15–20 minutes before carving. Serve with Gravy (see next recipe).

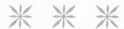

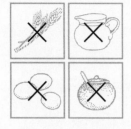

GRAVY

Serves 8

Adjust the herbs and spices to suit your taste. Each thickener produces a different texture.

1¾ cups low-sodium gluten-free chicken broth, divided	¼ teaspoon dried thyme leaves
½ cup strained drippings of turkey	¼ teaspoon poultry seasoning
¼ teaspoon salt	Thickener of your choice:
¼ teaspoon black pepper	Cornstarch: 2 tablespoons
¼ teaspoon ground sage	Rice flour: 4 tablespoons
	Tapioca flour: 6 tablespoons

1. Combine 1¼ cups of the broth and strained drippings in heavy saucepan, reserving ½ cup of the broth for step 2.
2. Place pan over medium-high heat; add seasonings. Stir thickener into ½ cup reserved broth, making thin paste. Gently whisk thickening mixture into pan, continuing to

whisk until mixture thickens and boils. Adjust consistency by adding more thickener or chicken broth. Remove from heat. Strain, if desired. Taste and adjust seasonings, if necessary.

Nutrition Information (per ¼-cup serving)
Calories 140 • Fat 14g • Protein 1g • Carbohydrates 2g • Cholesterol 14mg • Sodium 186mg • Fiber 0.5g

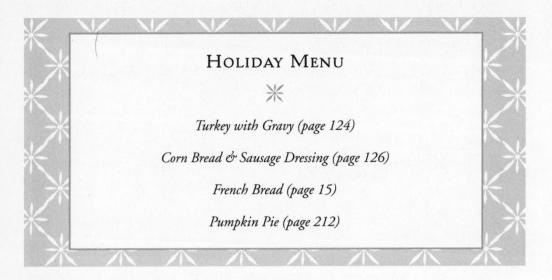

HOLIDAY MENU

※

Turkey with Gravy (page 124)

Corn Bread & Sausage Dressing (page 126)

French Bread (page 15)

Pumpkin Pie (page 212)

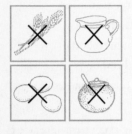

CORN BREAD & SAUSAGE DRESSING

Serves 16

This dressing is more like a bread pudding in texture—moist and tender. You'll need two batches of gluten-free corn bread if you use the recipe on page 31. Don't forget that you can make the gluten-free corn bread without eggs (page 32).

8 cups cubed gluten-free Corn Bread (page 31)	1 teaspoon celery seeds
½ pound gluten-free sausage	1 teaspoon dried oregano leaves
3 celery stalks, finely chopped	½ teaspoon salt (or to taste)
1 medium onion, finely chopped	½ teaspoon white pepper
3 teaspoons ground sage	2 cups gluten-free chicken broth
	2 cups 2% milk (cow, rice, or soy)

1. Preheat oven to 300°F. Layer corn bread cubes on large baking sheet. Bake until they are just lightly toasted, turning once during baking to assure even browning. Set aside.
2. Grease 13x9-inch nonstick baking pan. Set aside.
3. In heavy skillet over medium heat, brown sausage, celery, and onion. Drain well. In large bowl, combine corn bread cubes with remaining ingredients, stirring well. Turn into prepared baking pan. Bake for 30–40 minutes at 350°F until browned.

Nutrition Information (per serving)

Calories 335 • Fat 18g • Protein 11g • Carbohydrates 34g • Cholesterol 71mg • Sodium 725mg • Fiber 2g

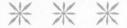

SOUTHWEST CHICKEN WITH PEACHES

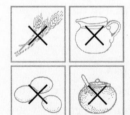

Serves 4

You've seen fancy restaurant dishes with multiple sauces, decoratively placed on the plate in exotic patterns. The secret? Fill empty plastic squeeze bottles such as those that contain mustard or ketchup with sauces like the balsamic syrup and chipotle sauce used in this recipe. You can refrigerate unused sauces for up to 1 week and use them creatively as accents to your entrées.

CHICKEN WITH SOUTHWEST MARINADE

¾ cup fresh lime juice

½ cup minced fresh cilantro

2 tablespoons olive oil

2 small garlic cloves, minced

2 teaspoons chili powder

2 teaspoons dried oregano

½ teaspoon cayenne pepper

½ teaspoon cumin powder

½ teaspoon salt

4 chicken breast halves

½ teaspoon cornstarch

2 teaspoons water

CHIPOTLE SAUCE

¼ cup boiling water

1 dried chipotle pepper

½ cup 2% milk (cow, rice, or soy)

1 teaspoon grated, peeled fresh
   gingerroot

¼ teaspoon salt

1 teaspoon fresh lemon or lime juice

1 teaspoon almond butter or cashew
   nut butter

BALSAMIC SYRUP

1 cup balsamic vinegar

1 teaspoon sugar

1 teaspoon ground coriander

PEACHES

2 firm, ripe unpeeled peaches

Fresh cilantro or parsley, and cherry
   tomatoes, for garnish

1. Assemble marinade ingredients (except chicken, cornstarch, and water) in shallow glass dish. Arrange chicken breasts, turn to coat thoroughly, cover, and refrigerate for 2–4 hours.
2. Grill chicken over coals or brown in a ridged skillet until done.
3. While chicken is cooking, heat marinade juices in small, heavy pan.
4. To make chipotle sauce, begin by bringing ¼ cup water to boiling. Place dried chipotle pepper in water and soak for 5–10 minutes. Finely chop chipotle pepper (wearing rubber gloves to protect hands) and reserve liquid. In food processor, combine chopped chipotle, soaking liquid, milk, gingerroot, salt, lemon (or lime) juice, and nut butter. Process until very smooth. Heat mixture in small, heavy saucepan over medium heat until thick.
5. To prepare balsamic syrup, bring balsamic vinegar, sugar, and coriander to boiling in small, heavy pan. Reduce heat to low; simmer until liquid is reduced to about ⅔ cup.

6. Cut peaches in half and remove pits. Place cut side down on grill. Brush with balsamic syrup; grill on both sides until grill marks are visible.

7. Just before serving, stir cornstarch into 2 teaspoons water to form paste. Stir paste into marinade over medium heat until slightly thickened. Place 2 tablespoons hot marinade in pool on plate. Place cooked chicken in pool.

8. Spoon chipotle sauce over each chicken. Drizzle balsamic syrup over chicken in decorative pattern. Add peach half. Garnish plate with cilantro or parsley and cherry tomatoes. Serve immediately.

Nutrition Information (per serving)

Calories 240 • Fat 10g • Protein 16g • Carbohydrates 24g • Cholesterol 37mg • Sodium 513mg • Fiber 2g

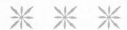

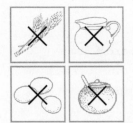

RASPBERRY-BASIL CHICKEN

Serves 6

Raspberry and basil complement each other in this truly delicious dish.

6 chicken breast halves	¼ teaspoon salt
⅓ cup fruit-only raspberry jam	¼ teaspoon black pepper
¼ cup pineapple juice	¼ teaspoon dry mustard
3 tablespoons wheat-free tamari soy sauce	¼ teaspoon chili powder
1 tablespoon rice vinegar or balsamic vinegar	¼ teaspoon curry powder
1 teaspoon dried basil leaves	1 small garlic clove, minced
	Fresh basil leaf, for garnish (optional)

1. Place chicken in greased, shallow baking dish.

2. Whisk together remaining ingredients except basil and pour half over chicken, reserving the other half. Marinate chicken for 30–45 minutes in refrigerator.

3. Preheat oven to 350°F. Bake chicken for 30–45 minutes, until done, basting occasionally. Heat remaining sauce and serve over chicken. Garnish with a sprig of fresh basil, if desired.

Nutrition Information (per serving)

Calories 110 • Fat 2g • Protein 14g • Carbohydrates 89g • Cholesterol 37mg • Sodium 635mg • Fiber 1g

Note: You can make your own dry mustard by grinding mustard seeds in a small coffee grinder.

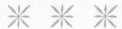

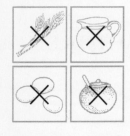

CHICKEN CACCIATORE

Serves 6

The aroma of this dish will fill your kitchen, inviting you and your family to a marvelous dining experience. Serve with hot cooked rice or pasta and a crunchy tossed salad. It is especially wonderful on a cold winter day.

4 chicken breast halves	2 tablespoons fresh lemon juice
1 tablespoon olive oil	2 teaspoons dried basil leaves
3 cups fresh mushrooms, halved	1 teaspoon sugar
1 small green bell pepper, chopped	1 teaspoon dried thyme leaves
1 large onion, sliced	½ teaspoon salt
1 garlic clove, minced	¼ teaspoon crushed red pepper flakes
½ cup dry red wine	¼ teaspoon black pepper
1 can (20 ounces) tomatoes, chopped	1 tablespoon cornstarch (if needed)
2 tablespoons tomato paste	2 tablespoons water (if needed)

1. In large, heavy skillet or Dutch oven, brown chicken on all sides in olive oil. Remove chicken from skillet and set aside.
2. Add mushrooms, green bell pepper, onion, and garlic to skillet. Cook until vegetables are tender. Add wine, bring to boiling, and simmer, uncovered, until liquid is nearly evaporated. Add undrained canned tomatoes, tomato paste, lemon juice, basil, sugar, thyme, salt, red pepper flakes, and black pepper.
3. Return chicken to skillet and simmer, uncovered, for 15 minutes—either on the stove top or in 350°F oven. If sauce is not thick enough, stir cornstarch with water and add to sauce, stirring until thickened.

Nutrition Information (per serving)
Calories 150 • Fat 4g • Protein 12g • Carbohydrates 15g • Cholesterol 24mg • Sodium 233mg • Fiber 3g

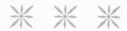

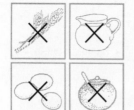

COQ AU VIN

Serves 4

A popular French dish, this is actually just chicken cooked in wine. It is an enticing blend of flavors, and the dish cooks slowly on its own, leaving you free to do other things. It's absolutely delicious and perfect for a fall or winter day.

1 slice bacon, uncooked
1 teaspoon olive oil
4 chicken breast halves
1 package (9 ounces) frozen pearl onions
3 garlic cloves, peeled
½ pound fresh mushrooms
1 cup low-sodium gluten-free chicken broth
½ cup dry red wine
1 teaspoon dried thyme leaves

1 teaspoon sugar or honey
1 teaspoon dried rosemary leaves
1 teaspoon paprika
½ teaspoon celery salt
½ teaspoon black pepper
1 pound small new potatoes
1 pound baby carrots
¼ teaspoon salt
1 tablespoon cornstarch (if needed)
2 tablespoons water (if needed)
½ cup chopped fresh parsley, for garnish

1. In heavy, ovenproof Dutch oven, brown bacon until crisp. Remove bacon and set aside. Add olive oil to pan and cook chicken until browned on all sides. Remove chicken and set aside.

2. In same Dutch oven, brown onions and garlic about 5 minutes. Add mushrooms and sauté 5 minutes more. Slowly pour in chicken broth and wine. Add thyme, sugar, rosemary, paprika, celery salt, and black pepper. Return chicken to pan and add potatoes and cooked bacon.

3. Bake, covered, 30 minutes at 400°F. Reduce heat to 350°F, add carrots and salt, and continue cooking another 30 minutes. Using slotted spoon, remove chicken and vegetables from Dutch oven. Keep warm on serving platter. If sauce does not need thickening, it may be served at this point by pouring over chicken and vegetables.

4. If sauce needs thickening, combine cornstarch and water to form paste. With Dutch oven over low-medium heat, stir in cornstarch mixture; boil until sauce thickens. Use more cornstarch for a thicker sauce.

5. Pour sauce over chicken and vegetables. Garnish with chopped parsley.

Nutrition Information (per serving)

Calories 320 • Fat 8g • Protein 20g • Carbohydrates 37g • Cholesterol 42mg • Sodium 688mg • Fiber 4g

CANDLELIGHT DINNER

Coq Au Vin (page 131)

Pasta

Roasted Fennel

Italian Bread Sticks (page 27)

Mixed Greens with Basic "Vinaigrette" (page 89)

Chocolate Cherry Cake (page 180)

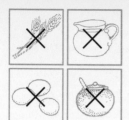

STIR~FRY LEMON CHICKEN

Serves 4

One of the secrets to attractive stir-fry dishes is to vary the shapes and colors of the various vegetables you use. For example, cut the carrots into ¼-inch ridged diagonals, the red or green bell peppers into long, ¼-inch-wide slices, and the green onions into 1-inch diagonals.

1 pound boneless, skinless chicken, cut into 1-inch pieces
¼ cup wheat-free tamari soy sauce
¼ cup fresh lemon juice
¼ cup water
1 tablespoon grated lemon zest
1 teaspoon honey or agave nectar
2 teaspoons crushed red pepper flakes
2 garlic cloves, minced
½ teaspoon ground ginger
1 tablespoon olive oil

3 green onions, diagonally cut into 1-inch pieces
2 medium carrots, diagonally cut into ½-inch pieces
½ cup red bell peppers, cut into ¼-inch strips
2 teaspoons cornstarch
2 cups hot cooked white rice
Additional green onions and lemon peel strips, for garnish (optional)

1. Place chicken in shallow, glass dish and set aside. Combine soy sauce, lemon juice, water, lemon zest, honey, crushed red pepper, garlic, and ginger. Pour half of marinade over chicken and reserve remaining half. Marinate chicken in the refrigerator for 30 minutes.
2. Drain chicken and discard marinade.
3. In heavy skillet over medium heat, sauté chicken in olive oil until lightly browned. Transfer meat to plate and cover with foil.
4. In same skillet, sauté onions, carrots, and red bell pepper until crisp-tender. Whisk cornstarch into reserved marinade. Stir into vegetables and stir-fry until thickened. Return chicken to skillet; bring to serving temperature.
5. Serve immediately over cooked rice. Garnish with additional chopped green onions and lemon strips, if desired.

Nutrition Information (per serving)

Calories 415 • Fat 7g • Protein 30g • Carbohydrates 57g* • Cholesterol 63mg • Sodium 999mg •
Fiber 3g

*Rice contributes 45g of the total 57g of carbohydrates per serving.

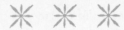

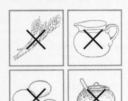

STIR-FRY ORANGE CHICKEN

Serves 4

This is a very beautiful, colorful dish. Get your family involved by having them chop the vegetables. You may use shrimp in place of chicken, if you wish.

SAUCE

½ cup low-sodium gluten-free
  chicken broth
½ cup fresh orange juice
3 tablespoons wheat-free tamari
  soy sauce
2 teaspoons rice vinegar

1 teaspoon sesame oil
1 tablespoon canola oil
1 teaspoon molasses
1 teaspoon sugar
3 tablespoons cornstarch

CHICKEN & VEGETABLES

1 teaspoon canola oil
4 boneless, skinless chicken breast
  halves, sliced diagonally into
  ½-inch pieces
3 tablespoons grated orange zest
1 garlic clove, minced
¼ teaspoon crushed red pepper flakes

1 cup sliced red and/or yellow bell
  peppers
1 cup snow peas, fresh or frozen
¼ cup carrots, diagonally cut into
  ½-inch pieces
¼ cup chopped fresh cilantro, packed
4 cups hot cooked white rice

1. Prepare sauce by whisking together sauce ingredients and set aside.
2. In large skillet or wok, heat oil over medium-high heat. Add chicken and cook until nicely browned.
3. Add orange zest, garlic, crushed red pepper, bell peppers, snow peas, and carrots. Sauté for 2–3 minutes.
4. Stir in sauce mixture and simmer for 4–5 minutes until mixture thickens and reduces slightly. Add cilantro. Serve over cooked rice.

Nutrition Information (per serving)
Calories 205 • Fat 6g • Protein 17g • Carbohydrates 64g* • Cholesterol 37mg • Sodium 810mg • Fiber 3g

*Rice contributes 44g of the total 64g of carbohydrates per serving.

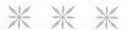

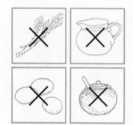

BARBECUED RIBS WITH 19TH-HOLE SAUCE

Serves 12

This is one of my favorite summertime dishes. Precooking the ribs makes them turn out deliciously tender and succulent.

8 pounds pork ribs
1 cup ketchup
½ cup molasses
½ cup orange juice
¼ cup red wine vinegar
2 tablespoons dried minced onion
2 tablespoons brown sugar or
  maple sugar
1 tablespoon mustard seeds
1 teaspoon chili powder
1 teaspoon crushed red pepper flakes

2 teaspoons paprika
1 teaspoon dried oregano leaves
½ teaspoon black pepper
½ teaspoon salt
1 bay leaf
1 garlic clove, minced
1 teaspoon grated orange zest
2 tablespoons olive oil
2 tablespoons Lea & Perrins
  Worcestershire sauce

1. Wrap ribs in aluminum foil and bake in 250°F oven for 3–4 hours. (This step can be done the day before. Refrigerate, covered.)
2. To make sauce, combine remaining ingredients in small saucepan. Bring to boiling, reduce heat to low, and simmer sauce for 10–15 minutes. Brush sauce on ribs as they cook on grill.

Nutrition Information (per serving)
Calories 690 • Fat 45g • Protein 42g • Carbohydrates 20g • Cholesterol 170mg • Sodium 270mg • Fiber 1g

NEIGHBORHOOD BLOCK PARTY

Barbecued Ribs with 19th-Hole Sauce (page 135)

Coleslaw

Potato Salad (page 103)

Garlic French Bread (page 16)

Double Chocolate Cherry Torte (page 183)

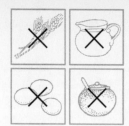

GRILLED PORK WITH ORANGE-ROSEMARY SAUCE

Serves 4

This dish can also be transformed into a last-minute quick dinner—if you skip marinating the pork in the sauce. For a smoother sauce, be sure to grate rather than chop the onion.

4 pork chops, 1¼ pounds

2 tablespoons molasses or sorghum syrup

½ cup fresh orange juice

1 teaspoon grated orange zest

2 teaspoons Dijon mustard

1 teaspoon olive oil

1 teaspoon balsamic vinegar

¼ teaspoon salt

¼ teaspoon black pepper

1 teaspoon crushed dried rosemary leaves

1 small garlic clove, minced

2 tablespoons grated fresh onion

1 teaspoon cornstarch

1 tablespoon water

Fresh rosemary sprigs, for garnish (optional)

1. Place pork chops in shallow dish or heavy-duty plastic freezer bag. Combine all sauce ingredients (molasses through onion) and pour over pork. Marinate for 6–8 hours. Remove pork, reserving marinade, and grill until done.

2. Meanwhile, while pork is cooking, bring marinade to boil in small saucepan over medium heat, reduce to low, and simmer for 5 minutes. Baste chops with the cooked sauce as they grill, if you wish.

3. Just before serving, mix cornstarch with water. Whisk into sauce, continuing to stir until mixture thickens. Remove from heat. Serve over pork and garnish with fresh rosemary sprigs, if desired.

Nutrition Information (per serving)
Calories 250 • Fat 8g • Protein 31g • Carbohydrates 13g • Cholesterol 90mg • Sodium 268mg • Fiber 1g

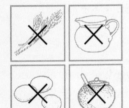

PORK FRIED RICE

Serves 4

This is a great way to use up leftover rice. It's quick and easy and the perfect answer when someone says, "Let's have Chinese tonight."

½ pound boneless pork, cut into
    ¼-inch-thick cubes
1 tablespoon canola oil
1 small onion, finely chopped
2 small garlic cloves, minced
1 large carrot, diagonally cut into
    ¼-inch pieces
½ cup chopped mushrooms
1 large egg, beaten (optional)

4 cups cooked white rice
2 tablespoons wheat-free tamari
    soy sauce
3 green onions, cut into ¼-inch pieces
½ cup snow peas
¼ pound (2 cups) bean sprouts
1 teaspoon sesame oil
½ teaspoon salt
¼ teaspoon black pepper

1. In wok or high-edged skillet, sauté pork cubes in oil until lightly browned and cooked through. Remove from pan.
2. Add onion and stir-fry until onion is translucent. Add garlic, carrot, and mushrooms; cook for 2 minutes. Add this mixture to cooked pork. Remove all ingredients from wok and set aside.
3. In wok, stir-fry egg (if using) and cook until set. Break up pieces using spatula. Add rice and all cooked ingredients to wok. Add soy sauce, green onions, snow peas, bean sprouts, oil, salt, and pepper. Stir to combine and bring to serving temperature. Serve immediately.

Nutrition Information (per serving)

Calories 330 • Fat 15g • Protein 17g • Carbohydrates 35g • Cholesterol 86mg • Sodium 890mg • Fiber 3g

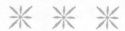

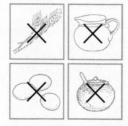

PORK MEDALLIONS WITH CHERRY SAUCE

Serves 6

This recipe is perfect for a weekend dinner, and you can prepare the rest of the meal while the pork is roasting.

2 pounds pork tenderloin
1 teaspoon black pepper
1 cup dried tart cherries
1 cup port wine or red grape juice, divided

1 teaspoon unsalted butter or canola oil
¼ cup balsamic vinegar
½ teaspoon dried marjoram leaves

1. Season pork chops with pepper. Roast in 325°F oven until thermometer registers 160°F (about 25 minutes per pound).

2. In small pan over medium heat, combine cherries and ⅓ cup of port wine. Bring to simmer. Turn off heat; let cherries soak for 15 minutes. Return mixture and remaining port wine to medium heat. Add remaining ingredients; boil to thicken. This sauce can be made ahead of time and reheated just before serving. Serve on sliced pork.

Nutrition Information (per serving)
Calories 360 • Fat 8g • Protein 43g • Carbohydrates 21g • Cholesterol 122mg • Sodium 91mg • Fiber 1g

WEEKEND DINNER

Pork Medallions with Cherry Sauce (page 139)

Rice Pilaf

Spinach Salad with Strawberries (page 104)

Steamed Vegetables

Frozen Tiramisu (page 218)

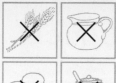
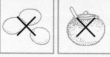

THAI PORK NOODLE BOWL

Serves 6

Why go out for Thai food when you can prepare this tasty dish right at home?

½ pound boneless pork, cut into
  ½-inch cubes
¼ cup chopped green onions
1 garlic clove, minced
1 tablespoon canola oil
½ cup chopped red bell pepper
¼ cup rice vinegar
3 tablespoons wheat-free tamari
  soy sauce
⅓ cup packed light brown sugar
  or maple sugar

4 teaspoons sweet paprika
1 teaspoon Reese's anchovy paste
¾ teaspoon cayenne pepper
¼ cup chopped fresh cilantro
2 cups mung bean sprouts
12 ounces rice noodles, cooked
¼ cup chopped cashews, for garnish
  (optional)

1. In large, heavy skillet over medium heat, sauté pork, green onions, and garlic in oil until pork is done.
2. Add bell pepper, vinegar, soy sauce, sugar, paprika, anchovy paste, and cayenne pepper to skillet and toss, along with cilantro, until hot.
3. Place bean sprouts and cooked noodles on plate. Top with meat mixture. Garnish with chopped cashews, if desired.

Nutrition Information (per serving)
Calories 260 • Fat 7g • Protein 25g • Carbohydrates 27g • Cholesterol 67mg • Sodium 487mg •
  Fiber 1g

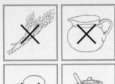
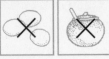

BAYOU RED BEANS & RICE

Serves 8

A slow cooker is an ideal way to cook the beans. Assemble the ingredients in the morning and let them cook all day. You'll be greeted with a wonderful aroma when you arrive home from work.

1 celery stalk, chopped

1 small yellow onion, chopped

3 garlic cloves, minced

1 teaspoon olive oil

1 pound dried red beans
   (not kidney beans)

1 teaspoon dried basil leaves

1 teaspoon crushed dried rosemary
   leaves

½ teaspoon dried oregano leaves

½ teaspoon dried thyme leaves

2 teaspoons salt

1 teaspoon black pepper

2 tablespoons packed light brown
   sugar or maple sugar

⅛ teaspoon cayenne pepper

2 bay leaves

¼ pound Canadian-style bacon,
   cut into 1-inch pieces

Water to cover beans

4 cups hot cooked white rice

1 tablespoon chopped fresh parsley,
   for garnish (optional)

1. In large, heavy saucepan over medium heat, sauté celery, onion, and garlic in olive oil until translucent.

2. Rinse and pick over beans to remove stones or debris. Add to saucepan along with basil, rosemary, oregano, thyme, salt, black pepper, sugar, cayenne pepper, bay leaves, and Canadian bacon.

3. Add enough water to cover beans and simmer over medium heat for 2 hours, or until beans are done. Serve over cooked rice. Garnish with parsley, if desired.

Nutrition Information (per serving)

Calories 220 • Fat 2g • Protein 9g • Carbohydrates 40g* • Cholesterol 7mg • Sodium 910mg •
   Fiber 6g

*Rice contributes 22g of the total 40g of carbohydrates per serving.

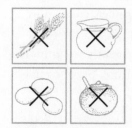

SWEET-AND-SOUR PORK

Serves 6

This is an old standby, but a real favorite. For the prettiest effect, be sure to vary the shapes of the vegetables. Cut the carrots into ¼-inch ridge diagonals, the bell peppers into ¼-inch-thick slices, and the onions into quarters.

MARINADE & PORK

1 tablespoon wheat-free tamari
   soy sauce

1 teaspoon ground ginger

1 tablespoon cornstarch

1 garlic clove, minced

1 tablespoon pineapple juice

1 pound boneless pork, cut into
   1-inch cubes

VEGETABLES & SAUCE

1 small onion, coarsely chopped

1 carrot, cut into ¼-inch-thick slices

1 tablespoon canola oil

½ cup chopped red bell pepper

1 small green bell pepper, chopped

1 can (8 ounces) pineapple chunks in juice

2 tablespoons brown sugar or maple sugar

3 tablespoons cider vinegar

1 tablespoon grated, peeled fresh gingerroot

2 tablespoons wheat-free tamari soy sauce

⅛ teaspoon white pepper

1 tablespoon tapioca flour

1 tablespoon water

4 cups hot cooked white rice

1. Combine marinade ingredients in bowl and add pork cubes to marinate.

2. In heavy skillet over medium heat, brown onion, carrots, and pork cubes in oil until lightly browned, stirring frequently. Remove from skillet and set aside.

3. Sauté red and green bell peppers 3 minutes, stirring frequently. Remove from skillet and set aside.

4. To skillet, add pineapple chunks (including juice and enough water to equal ⅔ cup liquid), sugar, vinegar, ginger, soy sauce, and pepper over medium heat. Stir together the tapioca flour and water until paste forms. Stir slowly into skillet, continuing to stir until mixture thickens slightly.

5. Return pork, onion, and carrots to skillet. Cover and simmer gently for minutes. Add red and green bell peppers and bring to serving temperature. Serve over hot cooked rice.

Nutrition Information (per serving)

Calories 390 • Fat 14g • Protein 18g • Carbohydrates 47g* • Cholesterol 52mg • Sodium 553mg • Fiber 2g

*Rice contributes 25g of the total 47g of carbohydrates per serving.

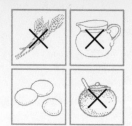

COCONUT SHRIMP

Serves 4

If eggs are inappropriate for your diet, dip the shrimp in the flour mixture only.

1 pound jumbo shrimp

½ cup cornstarch

½ cup shredded coconut

½ teaspoon garlic powder

½ teaspoon onion powder

½ teaspoon baking powder

½ teaspoon salt

¼ teaspoon cayenne pepper

2 large egg whites, beaten to foam

Oil, for frying

Orange marmalade, for dipping

1. Peel and clean shrimp, removing intestinal vein. To butterfly shrimp, use paring knife to open shrimp down the back without cutting all the way through. Press each shrimp flat and set aside.

2. In bowl, whisk together cornstarch, coconut, garlic and onion powders, baking powder, salt, and cayenne pepper.

3. In large bowl, whisk egg whites until they reach foamy texture. Heat enough cooking oil to cover shrimp in deep fryer or deep, heavy pot. Dip each shrimp in eggs, then in coconut-flour mixture. Fry shrimp in small batches, turning twice to assure even browning. Drain on paper towels. Continue with remaining shrimp. Serve with purchased orange marmalade as dip.

Nutrition Information (per serving)

Calories 285 • Fat 7g • Protein 19g • Carbohydrates 40g • Cholesterol 188mg • Sodium 525mg • Fiber 2g

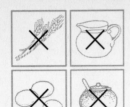

SHRIMP CREOLE

Serves 4

This dish makes an excellent weeknight dinner because it's so quick. Assemble the ingredients the night before to save time on extra-busy nights.

½ cup chopped onion

1 garlic clove, minced

½ cup chopped celery

1 tablespoon olive oil

1 can (16 ounces) peeled tomatoes

1 can (8 ounces) tomato sauce

1 tablespoon Lea & Perrins
  Worcestershire sauce

1 teaspoon salt

1 teaspoon sugar or honey

¾ teaspoon chili powder

½ teaspoon celery salt

⅛ teaspoon cayenne pepper

2 teaspoons cornstarch

1 tablespoon cold water

1 pound shrimp, peeled and deveined

½ cup chopped green bell pepper

4 cups hot cooked white rice

¼ cup chopped fresh parsley,
  for garnish

1. In large, heavy Dutch oven, sauté the onion, garlic, and celery in olive oil over medium heat until tender, but not brown. Add tomatoes, tomato sauce, Worcestershire sauce, salt, sugar, chili powder, celery salt, and cayenne pepper. Simmer, uncovered, for 30 minutes.

2. Mix cornstarch with cold water until smooth. Stir into sauce. Cook over medium heat, stirring, until bubbly. Add shrimp and green bell pepper. Cover and simmer on low heat for another 5 minutes.

3. To mold cooked rice, spray a Bundt pan or other decoratively shaped pan with cooking spray. Pack hot cooked rice in pan. It works better to fill pan all the way to the top, rather than using a larger pan that you only fill halfway. Turn out on serving plate.

4. For an even more decorative presentation, serve a colorful vegetable such as hot cooked green peas in the center hole (if using Bundt pan). Serve Shrimp Creole over hot cooked rice. Garnish with parsley.

Nutrition Information (per serving)

Calories 430 • Fat 7g • Protein 30g • Carbohydrates 62g* • Cholesterol 170mg • Sodium 13mg • Fiber 4g

*Rice contributes 45g of total 62g of carbohydrates per serving.

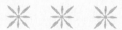

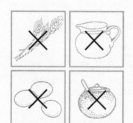

Paella

Serves 6

All you need with this dish is a tossed salad and bread. Serve it in a large, attractive dish—perhaps the one you cook it in. I cook mine in a large, flat copper pan that goes from oven to tabletop.

3 pounds chicken drumsticks	1 teaspoon Beau Monde seasoning
2 tablespoons olive oil	½ teaspoon crushed saffron threads
4 ounces Sausage (page 153)	1 teaspoon salt
½ cup chopped onion	¼ teaspoon black pepper
1 small tomato, chopped	3 cups low-sodium gluten-free
8 ounces shrimp, peeled and deveined	chicken broth
1 package (9 ounces) frozen artichoke	1½ cups uncooked white rice
hearts, or 1 can (16 ounces)	3 ounces pimientos (optional)
artichoke hearts	1 dozen mussels or clams on
1 garlic clove, minced	the shell
¼ cup chopped fresh parsley	8 ounces fish fillets (cod or perch)
1 teaspoon paprika	1 cup green peas

1. In large Dutch oven, brown chicken on all sides in olive oil. Remove from Dutch oven and set aside. Add sausage, onion, and tomato and cook until onion is lightly browned.

2. Return chicken to pan, and add shrimp and remaining ingredients except green peas. Cover and simmer for 30 minutes. (If using an ovenproof skillet, you may also place skillet in oven to cook.) Uncover, add green peas, and cook for another 5 minutes.

Nutrition Information (per serving)
Calories 680 • Fat 27g • Protein 59g • Carbohydrates 51g • Cholesterol 217mg • Sodium 1064mg • Fiber 6g

---

SEAFOOD DINNER

Paella (page 147)

Mixed Greens with Basic "Vinaigrette" (page 89)

Italian Bread Sticks (page 27) or French Bread (page 15)

Double Chocolate Cherry Torte (page 183)

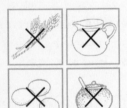

SPICY SHRIMP & PASTA

Serves 4

This beautiful dish is very attractive and colorful, with the contrast of the snow peas and red bell peppers against the pasta. If you like extra-spicy foods, increase the cayenne pepper a bit. Also, if you prefer not to use wine, you may use the same amount of chicken broth instead.

1 tablespoon canola oil

8 ounces snow peas, fresh or frozen

1 red bell pepper, cut into ¼-inch strips

1 medium garlic clove, minced

1 tablespoon tapioca flour

1 cup low-sodium gluten-free chicken broth, divided

½ cup dry white wine

½ teaspoon dried basil leaves

½ teaspoon paprika

½ teaspoon dried thyme leaves

¼ teaspoon cayenne pepper

¼ teaspoon black pepper

¼ teaspoon crushed red pepper flakes

1 pound medium-size shrimp, peeled and deveined

4 cups cooked gluten-free fettuccine or spaghetti

1 tablespoon chopped fresh parsley, divided, for garnish

½ cup grated Parmesan cheese (cow, rice, or soy), for garnish

1 teaspoon grated lemon zest, divided, for garnish

1. Place oil in large, heavy skillet. Over low-medium heat, sauté peas, bell pepper, and garlic for about 3 minutes, until vegetables are crisp-tender. Remove vegetables and set aside.

2. In same skillet, combine tapioca flour with 2 tablespoons of the chicken broth to form smooth paste. Then add wine and remaining chicken broth. Stir in basil, paprika, thyme, cayenne pepper, black pepper, and crushed red pepper. Bring mixture to boiling until slightly thickened.

3. Add shrimp. Reduce heat; cook for 5 minutes, or until shrimp are pink and curled. Return vegetables to skillet and cook for 1 minute longer. Remove from heat and cover to keep warm.

4. To serve, divide cooked pasta among 4 serving plates. Garnish with ½ tablespoon fresh parsley, sprinkle of Parmesan cheese, and ½ teaspoon lemon zest. Just before serving, toss shrimp mixture with remaining lemon zest and chopped parsley. Serve over hot noodles. Sprinkle with more Parmesan cheese, if desired.

Nutrition Information (per serving)

Calories 425 • Fat 10g • Protein 33g • Carbohydrates 47g • Cholesterol 171mg • Sodium 790mg • Fiber 5g

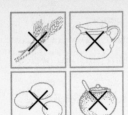

TUNA BURGERS WITH GRILLED PINEAPPLE SLICES

Serves 4

These burgers are an interesting change from ordinary hamburgers. Grilled pineapple slices add flavor, color, variety, and nutrients to any meal. If you're not using the outdoor barbecue grill, try using a ridged skillet on top of the range.

ORIENTAL SAUCE

1 cup pineapple juice or apple juice

½ cup rice vinegar or fresh lime juice

¼ cup wheat-free tamari soy sauce

¼ cup packed light brown sugar or maple sugar

¼ cup fresh lemon juice

1 teaspoon white pepper

1 teaspoon ground ginger

⅛ teaspoon ground allspice

½ teaspoon cornstarch

1 tablespoon cold water

TUNA BURGERS

1 pound fresh tuna steaks, or 3 cans (6 ounces each) gluten-free tuna in spring water

½ cup gluten-free bread crumbs

1 large egg, or ¼ cup Flax Mix (page 108)

1 tablespoon wheat-free tamari soy sauce

1 teaspoon dry mustard

½ teaspoon dried thyme leaves

½ teaspoon salt

½ teaspoon black pepper

GRILLED PINEAPPLE SLICES

1 can (16 ounces) pineapple slices

1 teaspoon canola oil

Dash paprika, for garnish

1. To make sauce, combine all sauce ingredients except cornstarch and cold water in small saucepan. Bring to boiling over medium heat, reduce to low, and simmer until liquid is reduced by half. Just before serving, combine cornstarch and water and stir until smooth. Add to sauce, stirring until mixture thickens slightly. Set aside.

2. While sauce cooks, begin to prepare burgers by grinding fresh tuna in food processor, or drain canned tuna. Combine with remaining burger ingredients and shape into 4 patties.
3. In large cast-iron skillet, nonstick skillet, or barbecue grill, cook tuna burgers on both sides.
4. Coat pineapple slices with oil. Grill for 3–5 minutes, turning when grill marks are visible on underside. Handle carefully so slices don't slip through grate, or use metal basket specially designed for grilling.
5. Serve burgers with sauce and pineapple slices. Garnish with dash of paprika.

Nutrition Information (per serving)
Calories 480 • Fat 12g • Protein 34g • Carbohydrates 62g • Cholesterol 88mg • Sodium 1728mg • Fiber 2g

Note: You can make your own dry mustard by grinding mustard seeds in a small coffee grinder.

FAMILY PICNIC

Tuna Burgers with Grilled Pineapple Slices (page 150)

Roasted Potatoes

Steamed Peas

Italian Bread Sticks (page 27)

Colorado Chocolate Chip Cookies (page 231)

Chocolate Cappuccino "Ice Cream" (page 240)

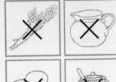

CHORIZO (MEXICAN SAUSAGE)

Makes 12 patties

Chorizo is a spicy sausage often served in Southwestern dishes.

1 pound ground round
2 pounds ground pork
3 garlic cloves, minced
⅓ cup vinegar
1 tablespoon paprika
2 teaspoons dried oregano leaves

1 teaspoon salt
1 teaspoon crushed red pepper flakes
1 teaspoon ground coriander
1 teaspoon ground cumin
½ teaspoon ground cloves

1. In large bowl, mix ground meats together. Add remaining ingredients and mix thoroughly. Shape into large ball or log. Chill.
2. Shape meat mixture into 12 patties, ½ inch thick and 2 inches in diameter, or 12 links, 3 inches long and ¾ inch wide.
3. In nonstick pan coated with cooking spray, fry patties until nicely browned on both sides.

Nutrition Information (per patty)
Calories 230 • Fat 15g • Protein 22g • Carbohydrates 1g • Cholesterol 64mg • Sodium 260mg • Fiber 0.5g

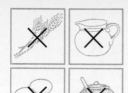

SAUSAGE

Serves 12

This tasty sausage makes a wonderful breakfast or add it to a spaghetti sauce for a tasty entrée.

1 pound ground round

1 pound ground pork

1 pound ground turkey

4 garlic cloves, minced

½ cup finely chopped onion

½ cup minced green bell pepper

½ cup minced red bell pepper

2 teaspoons chopped fresh cilantro

2 teaspoons ground cumin

2 teaspoons dried thyme leaves

2 teaspoons fennel seed

1 teaspoon salt

½ teaspoon crushed red pepper flakes

¼ teaspoon ground nutmeg

1. In large bowl, mix together all ingredients with your hands or large spatula. Shape meat into large ball or log. Refrigerate for 4 hours. Shape mixture in patties or meatballs. Place on baking sheet.
2. Bake at 350°F for 20–25 minutes, until browned.

Nutrition Information (per serving)

Calories 215 • Fat 13g • Protein 22g • Carbohydrates 2g • Cholesterol 66mg • Sodium 270mg • Fiber 0.5g

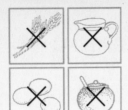

ORANGE-BEEF STIR-FRY

Serves 4

Looking for a change of pace? This tasty dish is different, easy to prepare, and looks great on your plate. Your family will love it.

1 cup fresh orange juice
¼ cup grated orange zest
1 tablespoon molasses or sorghum syrup
¼ cup wheat-free tamari soy sauce
1 tablespoon rice vinegar
2 tablespoons cornstarch
1 pound lean beef, sliced diagonally into ¼-inch slices
1 tablespoon canola oil

1 large garlic clove, minced
1 tablespoon grated, peeled fresh gingerroot
½ teaspoon crushed red pepper flakes
8 ounces broccoli florets, sliced
1 small red bell pepper, chopped
½ cup sliced green onions
4 cups hot cooked white rice

1. Combine orange juice, orange zest, molasses, soy sauce, rice vinegar, and cornstarch and set aside.
2. In large, heavy skillet or wok, brown meat in oil until lightly seared and no longer pink. Remove from pan and keep warm.
3. In same pan, cook garlic, ginger, crushed red pepper flakes, broccoli florets, and red bell pepper, stirring, over medium heat for 1 minute. Cover and cook for 1 more minute. Remove cover and add orange juice mixture to pan, stirring until mixture thickens. Return beef to pan, add chopped green onions, and bring to serving temperature. Serve over rice.

Nutrition Information (per serving)
Calories 410 • Fat 10g • Protein 32g • Carbohydrates 67g* • Cholesterol 66mg • Sodium 892mg • Fiber 4g

*Rice contributes 44g of total 67g of carbohydrates per serving.

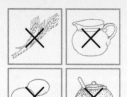

CHINESE HOT-SOUR SOUP

Serves 4

If you don't use the egg, the soup might not be quite as thick, but it will still be delicious. To julienne vegetables, simply cut them into thin matchsticks.

4 cups low-sodium gluten-free
  beef broth
2 green onions, thinly sliced, divided
1 small carrot, julienned
1 tablespoon grated, peeled fresh
  gingerroot
½ teaspoon white pepper
1 teaspoon canola oil
1 cup sliced fresh mushrooms

½ cup tofu, cut into ¼-inch cubes
1 cup diced cooked dark turkey
⅛ teaspoon cayenne pepper
1 teaspoon wheat-free fish sauce
  (optional)
1 tablespoon cornstarch or arrowroot
2 tablespoons rice vinegar or fresh
  lemon juice
1 egg white, well beaten (optional)

1. In large saucepan, combine beef broth, green onions (reserve 2 tablespoons for garnish), carrot, ginger, and white pepper. Bring to boiling over high heat, then lower heat and simmer for 15 minutes.
2. In medium skillet, sauté mushrooms in cooking oil over high heat for about 1 minute. Add to beef stock, along with tofu, turkey, cayenne, and fish sauce (if using).
3. In small bowl, dissolve cornstarch in vinegar. Add to soup and stir about 1 minute, until thickened.
4. Remove soup from heat and, stirring constantly, slowly pour in beaten egg white (if using). Cook until egg is done. Taste and adjust seasonings, adding more vinegar or white pepper, if desired. Ladle soup into 4 serving bowls. Garnish with reserved sliced green onions.

Nutrition Information (per serving)
Calories 165 • Fat 7g • Protein 24g • Carbohydrates 12g • Cholesterol 30mg • Sodium 582mg •
  Fiber 3g

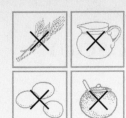

SPAGHETTI SAUCE & MEATBALLS

Serves 12

I've been making this thick, hearty low-fat sauce for more than twenty-five years, and even though we've tried several others, it remains our favorite. A slow cooker works best.

1 can (48 ounces) tomato juice

3 cans (6 ounces each) tomato paste

3 tablespoons dried parsley flakes

3 tablespoons granulated sugar, or
   1 tablespoon fructose powder

2 tablespoons dried basil leaves

1 tablespoon dried rosemary leaves

2 bay leaves

2 teaspoons dried oregano leaves

2 teaspoons salt

½ teaspoon black pepper

¼ cup grated Romano or Parmesan
   cheese (optional)

8 ounces Sausage, made into
   meatballs (page 153)

In large slow cooker, combine all ingredients, except sausage, mixing well. Cook all day on low-medium heat. Stir occasionally. Serve with meatballs and your favorite pasta.

Nutrition Information (per ¾-cup serving)
Calories 160 • Fat 9g • Protein 6g • Carbohydrates 18g • Cholesterol 15mg • Sodium 553mg •
   Fiber 3g

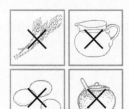

FRESH TOMATO-BASIL SAUCE WITH PASTA

Serves 4

Choose the most flavorful tomatoes you can find for this easy, fresh-tasting sauce.

4 plum tomatoes
2 large garlic cloves, minced
¼ cup extra-virgin olive oil, divided
½ teaspoon salt
¼ teaspoon black pepper

½ cup chopped fresh basil,
    or 2 tablespoons dried basil leaves
4 cups hot cooked gluten-free pasta
¼ cup grated Parmesan cheese (cow,
    rice, or soy), for garnish

1. Dip tomatoes in boiling water. Peel, quarter, and seed tomatoes.
2. In large bowl, crush tomatoes with potato masher. Drain again and reserve juice for another use.

3. In medium-sized, nonreactive pan, sauté garlic in 1 tablespoon of oil over medium heat for 2 minutes. Add tomatoes, salt, pepper, basil, and remaining oil. Simmer gently on low heat for 15 minutes, uncovered. Serve with pasta and garnish with Parmesan cheese.

Nutrition Information (per serving)

Calories 190 • Fat 16g • Protein 4g • Carbohydrates 9g • Cholesterol 5mg • Sodium 423mg • Fiber 2g

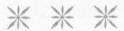

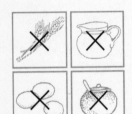

PAD THAI

Serves 4

This dish sounds difficult, but it's actually quite easy. Egg-sensitive people can simply omit the eggs. To julienne means to cut into thin, matchstick shapes.

8 ounces rice noodles, uncooked

2 quarts boiling water

2 teaspoons salt

¼ cup fresh lemon or lime juice

1 tablespoon wheat-free fish sauce (optional)

¼ cup wheat-free tamari soy sauce

1 tablespoon brown sugar or honey

¼ teaspoon crushed red pepper flakes

1 tablespoon sesame oil or olive oil

1 pound shrimp, peeled and deveined

1 cup snow peas

¼ cup julienned red bell pepper

½ cup sliced green onions

2 large garlic cloves, minced

2 large eggs, lightly beaten (optional)

2 cups bean sprouts

¼ cup chopped cashews

½ cup chopped fresh cilantro, divided

1. This dish cooks quickly, so have all ingredients assembled beforehand. Cook rice noodles in boiling water with salt. Drain thoroughly.

2. Meanwhile, while noodles are cooking, in small bowl combine lemon juice, fish sauce (if using), soy sauce, sugar, and crushed red pepper. Set aside.

3. Heat oil in wok or heavy skillet. Sauté shrimp, snow peas, red bell pepper, green onions, and garlic for 2–4 minutes over medium heat until shrimp turn pink. Add eggs (if using) and continue stirring until eggs are cooked. Add cooked noodles and lemon juice mixture and heat, stirring constantly, another 2–3 minutes.

4. Just before serving, stir in bean sprouts, cashews, and half of the cilantro. Garnish with additional nuts and remaining cilantro, if desired.

Nutrition Information (per serving)
Calories 295 • Fat 10g • Protein 26g • Carbohydrates 26g • Cholesterol 240mg • Sodium 1220mg • Fiber 3g

✳ ✳ ✳

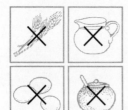

PASTA SALAD

Serves 4

Pasta salad is a great choice for those hot summer days when you don't want to be anywhere near a stove. Make this the night before and chill it. Bring to room temperature before serving.

2 cups gluten-free penne pasta (uncooked)	¼ teaspoon *each* salt and pepper
¼ cup olive oil	1 cup snow peas, blanched
¼ cup red wine vinegar	1 cup broccoli flowerets, blanched
2 tablespoons fresh lemon juice	1 small red bell pepper, chopped
1 tablespoon dried basil leaves	¼ cup pitted black olives, halved
1 teaspoon Dijon mustard	¼ cup toasted pine nuts
1 small garlic clove, minced	¼ cup grated Parmesan cheese (cow, rice, or soy) (optional)

1. Cook pasta in boiling, salted water. Drain and chill.

2. Meanwhile, whisk together oil, vinegar, lemon juice, basil, mustard, garlic, salt, and pepper.

3. Combine remaining ingredients in large bowl. Add cooked pasta. Toss with dressing. Chill.

Nutrition Information (per serving)

Calories 495 • Fat 22g • Protein 10g • Carbohydrates 65g • Cholesterol 5mg • Sodium 402mg • Fiber 2.5g

HOT SUMMER DAYS

Pasta Salad (page 159)

French Bread (page 15) or Italian Bread Sticks (page 27)

Your favorite frozen sherbet

Chocolate Cherry Cookies (page 227)

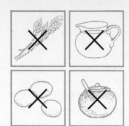

PIZZA SAUCE
& PIZZA CRUST

Serves 6

This is possibly my favorite recipe in the entire book. Why? Because pizza is the food we really miss when going on a gluten-free diet. I know you'll like this recipe as much as I do.

PIZZA SAUCE

1 can (8 ounces) tomato sauce

1½ teaspoons sugar or honey

½ teaspoon dried oregano leaves

½ teaspoon dried basil leaves

½ teaspoon crushed dried rosemary
   leaves

½ teaspoon fennel seed

½ teaspoon salt

¼ teaspoon garlic powder

Toppings of your choice

PIZZA CRUST

1 tablespoon active dry yeast

⅔ cup brown-rice flour

½ cup tapioca flour

2 teaspoons xanthan gum

1 teaspoon unflavored gelatin powder

1 teaspoon Italian seasoning

½ teaspoon sugar or honey

½ teaspoon salt

¾ cup warm milk (cow, rice, or soy)
   (110°F)

1 teaspoon olive oil

1 teaspoon cider vinegar

Extra rice flour, for sprinkling

1. Combine all sauce ingredients in small saucepan. Bring to boiling over medium heat. Reduce heat to low; simmer for 15 minutes while crust is being assembled. Makes about 1 cup.

2. Preheat oven to 425°F. Grease 12-inch pizza pan or baking sheet. In medium mixer bowl using regular beaters (not dough hooks), blend yeast, flours, xanthan gum, gelatin powder, Italian seasoning, sugar, and salt on low speed. Add warm milk, oil, and vinegar.

3. Beat on high speed for 2 minutes. Dough will resemble soft bread dough. If dough is too stiff, add water 1 tablespoon at a time. Put mixture on prepared pan. Liberally

sprinkle rice flour on dough, then press dough into pan, continuing to sprinkle dough with flour to prevent sticking to your hands. Make edges thicker to hold toppings.

4. Bake crust for 10 minutes. Remove from oven. Top with sauce and your preferred toppings. Bake for another 20–25 minutes, or until top is nicely browned. Cut into 6 slices.

Nutrition Information (per serving, crust only)
Calories 155 • Fat 1.5g • Protein 4g • Carbohydrates 33g • Cholesterol 1mg • Sodium 635mg • Fiber 3g

TIPS FOR THE PERFECT PIZZA

PIZZA PANS

Use nonstick, noninsulated metal pans for best results. Perforated pizza pans are not recommended for the first 10 minutes of baking because the unbaked dough falls through the perforations. However, once the pizza crust has baked for 10 minutes (prior to placing the toppings on it), you may slide the crust onto a perforated pan and continue baking as directed. Also, perforated pans work fine for reheating a whole pizza or pizza slices.

Some people have success using baking stones; others do not. The problem is that the wet, sticky dough tends to stick to the stone, making cleanup difficult. If you're determined to use the stone, sprinkle with cornmeal first or use parchment paper. Also, rather than patting the dough onto a preheated stone and burning yourself, pat it onto a cold stone. Then place in preheated oven. You'll need a peel (flat, wide wooden "spatula") to remove the pizza from the stone, or some stones have built-in carriers. The stone will be very hot.

Another idea is to bake the pizza on a nonstick pan for the first 10 minutes. Remove from the oven, top with toppings, and slide it onto a heated pizza stone in the oven. Once again, a wooden peel will reduce the chances of burned fingers.

WOOD-FIRED OR GRILLED PIZZAS

Yes, you can cook this pizza on a grill—just like in the restaurants. Bake the crust on a pizza pan in the oven for 10 minutes, as directed above. Top with toppings; transfer to a barbecue grill, using large spatulas or a wooden peel, if you have one. I use a gas grill with two temperature controls, placing the pizza over low heat on one side and keeping the other side at medium temperature. Close the lid and cook (peeking occasionally) for about 10 minutes, or until cheese is melted. The cheese won't brown as much as in the oven because there is no direct heat from above.

FREEZING

You may freeze the pizza crust after it has baked for 10 minutes. Or freeze the entire pizza after it has been topped with your favorite toppings and baked for 20 minutes. Be sure to cool thoroughly, then wrap tightly with aluminum foil before placing in the freezer. Some people prepare several pizza crusts; if so, bake them for 10 minutes and then freeze them, using them like the commercial pizza crusts you find in supermarkets. Defrost in the refrigerator. Microwaving may produce a slightly soggy crust.

STORING LEFTOVERS

Leftover pizza may be frozen (see Freezing above). Or wrap cooled pizza tightly and store in refrigerator for up to 2 days. Reheat in a low-medium hot skillet (with loose lid) on the stove.

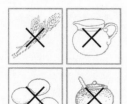

PIZZA MIX

Makes four 12-inch pizza crusts. Each pizza crust serves 6 for a total of 24.

Keep this mix on hand for quick meals.

2⅔ cups brown rice flour	4 teaspoons xanthan gum
2 cups tapioca flour	4 teaspoons unflavored gelatin powder
½ cup dry milk powder, nondairy milk powder, or almond flour	4 teaspoons Italian seasoning
	2 teaspoons salt

Combine all ingredients in airtight container and store in dark, dry place. To make one 12-inch pizza, place 1⅓ cups of dry mixture in medium bowl. Add 1 tablespoon active dry yeast, ¾ cup warm water (110°F), ½ teaspoon sugar (or ¼ teaspoon honey), 1 teaspoon olive oil, and 1 teaspoon cider vinegar. Mix with electric mixer on high speed for 3 minutes. Follow directions for Pizza Crust on page 161.

Nutrition Information (per serving, crust only)
Calories 100 • Fat .5g • Protein 2.5g • Carbohydrates 23g • Cholesterol 0mg • Sodium 190mg •
   Fiber 1g

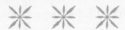

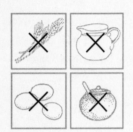

DAIRY-FREE, TOMATO-FREE PESTO PIZZA

Serves 6

Pizza Crust (page 161)
¾ cup pesto
**2 cups vegetables of your choice (sliced mushrooms, chopped
   pitted black olives, diced onion, red bell pepper, or other)**

1. Prepare pizza crust. Remove from oven and brush with pesto.
2. Sauté vegetables in skillet over medium heat until limp. Spread toppings over pizza. Bake for 15–20 minutes, or until desired doneness.

Nutrition Information (per serving of toppings)
Calories 260 • Fat 23g • Protein 8g • Carbohydrates 7mg • Cholesterol 13mg • Sodium 458mg •
   Fiber 1g

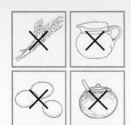

SUN-DRIED TOMATO & OLIVE PIZZA

Serves 6

Pizza Crust (page 161)
½ cup chopped sun-dried tomatoes
½ cup chopped pitted black olives
1 to 2 teaspoons dried oregano or basil leaves (or to taste)

Prepare pizza crust and remove from oven. Top with sun-dried tomatoes, black olives, and herbs. Bake at 425°F for 15–20 minutes.

Nutrition Information (per serving of toppings)
Calories 250 • Fat 22g • Protein 8g • Carbohydrates 7g • Cholesterol 13mg • Sodium 455mg • Fiber 1g

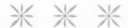

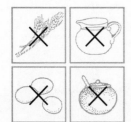

SPICY FETTUCCINE WITH BASIL

Serves 4

So simple to make and so impressive and tasty, this is the perfect entrée for a meatless meal. If you absolutely must have meat, try adding shrimp or cubed chicken.

½ cup extra-virgin olive oil, divided
2 large garlic cloves, minced
½ teaspoon crushed red pepper flakes
3 cups uncooked gluten-free fettuccine

6 quarts boiling, salted water
2 teaspoons dried basil leaves
⅓ cup gluten-free bread crumbs, toasted

½ cup grated Parmesan cheese
(cow, rice, or soy)

¼ cup chopped fresh parsley, for
garnish

4 plum tomatoes, finely chopped, for
garnish

1 lemon, cut into 4 wedges, for
garnish

1. Heat 1 tablespoon of oil in medium skillet over low heat. Sauté garlic and crushed
   red pepper for 2–3 minutes, stirring frequently. Set aside.
2. Cook fettucine in water about 2–3 minutes, until al dente. Drain, leaving ⅓ cup hot
   water in pot. Return pasta to pot; remove pot from heat. Add garlic mixture, remaining oil, basil, bread crumbs, and Parmesan cheese and toss gently. Garnish with
   chopped tomatoes, parsley, and lemon wedges. Serve immediately.

Nutrition Information (per serving)
Calories 500 • Fat 32g • Protein 8g • Carbohydrates 47g • Cholesterol 10mg • Sodium 333mg •
Fiber 3g

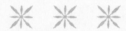

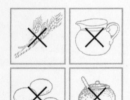

COLORADO CHILI

Serves 6

Cook this hearty dish in a slow cooker. If the chili thickens too much as it cooks, add
a bit of water.

1 pound ground round

1 cup finely chopped onion

1 can (15 ounces) pinto or
kidney beans

1 can (15 ounces) canned tomatoes

2 teaspoons chili powder

1 teaspoon salt

½ teaspoon ground allspice

½ teaspoon ground cumin

½ teaspoon ground coriander

¼ teaspoon ground cloves

¼ teaspoon ground cinnamon

Water (if too thick)

Chopped green onions, shredded
cheese, and fresh chopped cilantro,
for garnish

In large Dutch oven or skillet, combine ground round and chopped onion and cook over medium heat until browned. Add remaining ingredients, cover, and simmer for 2 hours. Or cook in slow cooker for 4–6 hours on low heat. Add more water if mixture becomes too thick. Serve with crackers and various garnishes—green onions, shredded cheese, and chopped fresh cilantro.

Nutrition Information (per serving)
Calories 210 • Fat 7g • Protein 20g • Carbohydrates 16g • Cholesterol 28mg • Sodium 466mg • Fiber 5g

---

SUPER BOWL PARTY

Colorado Chili (page 166)

Corn Bread with Green Chiles (page 31)

*Platter of ready-to-eat fresh vegetables
(baby carrots, celery, broccoli, radishes)*

Colorado Chocolate Chip Cookies (page 231)

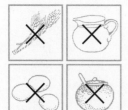

GREEN CHILE STEW

Serves 4

This hearty Southwestern dish makes an especially good Sunday night supper.

1 pound lean pork, cut into
  1-inch cubes
½ cup chopped onion

2 carrots, cut in ½-inch pieces
1 tablespoon olive oil
1 can (4 ounces) diced green chiles

3 cups low-sodium gluten-free
  beef broth
2 medium white potatoes, diced
4 plum tomatoes, diced
1 large garlic clove, minced
½ teaspoon ground cumin

½ teaspoon ground coriander
½ teaspoon dried oregano leaves
½ teaspoon salt
¼ teaspoon black pepper
½ cup chopped fresh cilantro

In heavy Dutch oven, brown pork, onion, and carrots in olive oil over medium heat until lightly browned. Add remaining ingredients except cilantro and simmer, covered, for 1 hour. Or, transfer mixture to slow cooker and simmer all day on Low. Add cilantro just before serving.

Nutrition Information (per serving)
Calories 340 • Fat 16g • Protein 26g • Carbohydrates 25g • Cholesterol 72mg • Sodium 480mg • Fiber 4g

MEXICAN MEAL

Green Chile Stew (page 167)

Corn Bread with Green Chiles (page 31)

Mexican Rice

Mexican Chocolate Cake (page 175)

DESSERTS

What's more perfect after a satisfying meal than a wickedly decadent chocolate brownie, or hearty cherry cobbler, or a thick, chewy cookie? Sure, they satisfy your sweet tooth, but desserts also create an opportunity to establish rituals—such as baking your child's favorite birthday cake every year, making an apple dish with the first hint of fall, or making homemade ice cream on a scorching summer day. You'll love these fabulous desserts because they don't let sensitivities to wheat, dairy, eggs, or cane sugar spoil the fun.

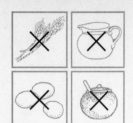

APPLESAUCE SPICE CAKE

Serves 10

Think of a crisp, fall day with the aroma of this cake in your kitchen. Wonderful! This recipe is perfect for the smaller 6-cup Bundt pan.

1 cup Flour Blend (page 276)

1½ teaspoons baking soda

1½ teaspoons baking powder

1 teaspoon ground cinnamon

1 teaspoon unflavored gelatin powder

½ teaspoon xanthan gum

½ teaspoon salt

½ teaspoon ground cloves

¼ teaspoon ground nutmeg

¼ teaspoon ground allspice

½ cup chopped walnuts

½ cup currants or dark raisins

⅓ cup butter or margarine, or ¼ cup canola oil

⅔ cup packed light brown sugar or maple sugar

2 large eggs, or ½ cup soft silken tofu

½ cup applesauce

1 tablespoon vinegar

1. Preheat oven to 350°F. Grease 6-cup nonstick Bundt cake pan.
2. Sift dry ingredients together (flour through allspice). Toss walnuts and currants with 2 tablespoons of the dry ingredients.
3. In large mixer bowl, cream butter, sugar, eggs or tofu, applesauce, and vinegar until thoroughly blended and very smooth. Slowly add dry ingredients, mixing just until combined. Fold in nuts and currants.
4. Transfer to prepared pan and bake for 25–30 minutes. Cool in pan for 5–10 minutes. Remove cake to wire rack and cool completely.

Nutrition Information (per serving)
Calories 230 • Fat 8g • Protein 3g • Carbohydrates 39g • Cholesterol 36mg • Sodium 438mg • Fiber 1g

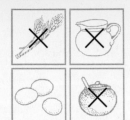

BASIC CAKE

Serves 12

This is an all-purpose basic cake that you can use for many occasions. For a white cake, use 3 egg whites rather than 2 whole eggs. For an egg-free version, see page 172.

⅓ cup butter or margarine, or ¼ cup
    canola oil
1 cup granulated sugar or fructose
    powder
2 large eggs, or 3 egg whites
1 tablespoon grated lemon zest
1½ cups Flour Blend (page 276)
1 teaspoon xanthan gum

½ teaspoon baking powder
½ teaspoon baking soda
¼ teaspoon salt
¾ cup buttermilk, or 2 teaspoons
    vinegar or lemon juice and enough
    nondairy milk to equal ¾ cup
1 teaspoon vanilla extract

1. Preheat oven to 325°F. Grease two 8-inch round nonstick baking pans and line with parchment paper or waxed paper. Or grease two 5x3-inch nonstick loaf pans.
2. Using electric mixer and large mixer bowl, cream butter and sugar on medium speed until thoroughly blended. Mix in eggs and lemon zest on low speed until blended.
3. In medium bowl, sift together flours, xanthan gum, baking powder, baking soda, and salt. In another medium bowl, combine buttermilk and vanilla.
4. On low speed, beat dry ingredients into butter mixture, alternating with buttermilk, beginning and ending with dry ingredients. Mix just until combined. Spoon batter equally into prepared pans and smooth tops.
5. Bake 8-inch cakes for about 30–35 minutes, small loaves for 30–40 minutes, or until tops are golden brown and a wooden pick inserted in center comes out clean. Cool cake in pans for 5 minutes, then remove from pans, remove paper, and cool on wire rack.

Nutrition Information (per serving)
Calories 230 • Fat 6g • Protein 3g • Carbohydrates 45g • Cholesterol 44mg • Sodium 189mg •
    Fiber 0.5g

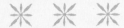

Variation

Lemon Poppy Seed Cake: Increase lemon zest to 2 tablespoons; add 2 tablespoons poppy seeds. Bake as directed.

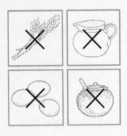

BASIC CAKE WITHOUT EGGS

Serves 12

This cake was designed for people who don't want to eat eggs. It can be baked as cupcakes, a layer cake, or used for any dessert that requires a basic cake. To save time, you can mix the dry ingredients up to 3 months ahead of time and add the liquid ingredients when you're ready to bake.

1¾ cups Flour Blend (page 276)
2¼ teaspoons baking powder
½ teaspoon xanthan gum
¼ teaspoon salt
¾ cup granulated sugar or fructose powder

½ cup (1 stick) butter or margarine, or ⅓ cup canola oil
½ cup soft silken tofu
2 teaspoons vanilla extract
Grated zest of 1 lemon
½ cup boiling water

1. Preheat oven to 350°F. Grease 11x7-inch nonstick baking pan (or two 5x3-inch nonstick loaf pans—or other pan sizes, see below). (This cake rises better in smaller pans.) Sift together flours, baking powder, xanthan gum, and salt. Set aside.
2. In food processor, process sugar, butter (at room temperature), tofu, vanilla, and lemon zest until completely smooth and glossy. Add boiling water and process until completely mixed. Add flour mixture and process until smooth. Scrape down sides of bowl with spatula, if necessary.

3. Spoon batter into prepared pan(s). Bake 11x7-inch cake for 25–30 minutes, small loaves for 30–40 minutes, or until tops are firm. Cake will not brown very much. Remove from oven and cool 10 minutes before removing from pan(s). Cool completely before cutting.

Nutrition Information (per serving)
Calories 200 • Fat 9g • Protein 4g • Carbohydrates 28g • Cholesterol 0mg* • Sodium 154mg • Fiber 0.5g

Variations

Cupcakes: Bake 12 standard-size cupcakes for 20–25 minutes, or until tops are firm.

Layer Cake: Grease, then line two 8- or 9-inch round nonstick cake pans with waxed paper or parchment paper; grease again. Spread batter evenly in pans; bake at 350°F for 25–30 minutes, or until tops are firm. Cool cake for 10 minutes before removing from pans. Cool on wire rack.

*Butter adds 20mg of cholesterol per serving.

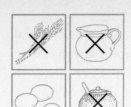

BASIC CHOCOLATE CAKE

Serves 12

This basic chocolate cake is extremely versatile and will become one of your favorites. It makes a somewhat small, but virtually fail-safe cake. For an egg-free version, see page 175.

1¼ cups Flour Blend
  (page 276)
½ cup unsweetened cocoa powder
  (not Dutch process)
1 teaspoon xanthan gum
1 teaspoon baking soda
¾ teaspoon salt

1 cup packed light brown sugar
  or maple sugar
2 teaspoons vanilla extract
½ cup 2% milk (cow, rice, or soy)
½ cup (1 stick) butter or margarine
1 large egg
¾ cup warm coffee or water (110°F)

1. Preheat oven to 350°F. Grease 9-inch round, 9-inch square, or 11x7-inch nonstick baking pan.
2. Place all ingredients except coffee in large mixer bowl and blend with electric mixer. Add coffee and mix until thoroughly blended. Pour into prepared pan; bake for 30–35 minutes, or until wooden pick inserted in center of cake comes out clean. Cool completely before cutting.

Nutrition Information (per serving)
Calories 220 • Fat 9g • Protein 2g • Carbohydrates 35g • Cholesterol 57mg • Sodium 330mg • Fiber 1.5g

Variations

Cupcakes: Bake 12 cupcakes for 20–25 minutes, or until wooden pick inserted in center comes out clean.

Layer Cake: Double recipe (increase baking soda to 1¼ teaspoons) and bake in two 9-inch round nonstick cake pans for 35–40 minutes, or two 8-inch round nonstick cake pans for 25–30 minutes, or until wooden pick inserted in center comes out clean. Also, first grease and line with waxed paper or parchment paper; then grease again for easier cake removal.

Mexican Chocolate Cake: Add 1½ teaspoons almond extract and 1 tablespoon ground cinnamon in step 2. Bake as directed.

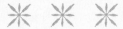

BASIC CHOCOLATE CAKE WITHOUT EGGS

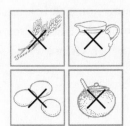

Serves 12

This version can be used just like the chocolate cake recipe on page 174. If you prefer a larger cake, double the recipe but only use 2½ teaspoons baking powder.

1¼ cups Flour Blend (page 276)
½ cup unsweetened cocoa powder (not Dutch process)
2¼ teaspoons baking soda
½ teaspoon xanthan gum
½ teaspoon salt
¾ cup packed light brown sugar or maple sugar

¼ cup (½ stick) butter or margarine, at room temperature, or canola oil
½ cup soften silken tofu
2 teaspoons vanilla extract
⅔ cup hot coffee or water (115°F)

1. Preheat oven to 350°F. Grease a 9-inch round or 9-inch square nonstick baking pan. Combine flours, cocoa, baking soda, xanthan gum, and salt. Set aside.
2. In food processor, process sugar, butter or oil, tofu, and vanilla until very smooth. Add hot coffee or water and blend until completely mixed. Add flour mixture and blend at low speed until smooth.
3. Spoon batter into prepared pan. Bake for 25–30 minutes, or until top is firm and wooden pick inserted in center comes out clean. Remove from oven. Cool for 5 minutes before removing from pan.

Nutrition Information (per serving)
Calories 170 • Fat 5g • Protein 2g • Carbohydrates 32g • Cholesterol 10mg • Sodium 200mg • Fiber 1.5g

Variations

Cupcakes: Bake 12 cupcakes 20–25 minutes, or until wooden pick inserted in center comes out clean.

Layer Cake: Double recipe (use 1 tablespoon baking soda) and bake in two 9-inch round nonstick baking pans for 30–35 minutes, or two 8-inch round nonstick baking pans for 25–30 minutes, or until wooden pick inserted in center comes out clean. Also, first grease and then line the pans with waxed paper or parchment paper. Grease waxed paper or parchment for easier cake removal.

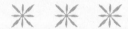

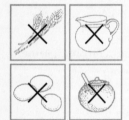

BLACK FOREST BROWNIE TORTE

Serves 12

If you love chocolate and cherry, you'll love this dessert. You can use commercial cherry pie filling or make your own using the recipe on page 248.

1¼ cups Flour Blend (page 276)
½ cup unsweetened cocoa powder
   (not Dutch process)
1 teaspoon baking powder
1 teaspoon xanthan gum
½ teaspoon salt

¼ cup (½ stick) butter or margarine,
   at room temperature, or canola oil
½ cup granulated sugar
½ cup packed light brown sugar or
   maple sugar
1 large egg*

2 teaspoons vanilla extract

½ cup hot water or coffee (115°F)

Cherry Pie Filling (page 248), or

    1 can (22 ounces) cherry pie filling

Whipped Topping (page 203)

1 cup Chocolate Syrup (page 198)

1. Preheat oven to 350°F. Grease two 8-inch round nonstick baking pans. Line with parchment paper or waxed paper and grease again.
2. Stir together flours, cocoa, baking powder, xanthan gum, and salt. In large mixer bowl, beat butter and sugars with electric mixer on medium speed until well combined.
3. Add egg and vanilla; beat until well combined. With mixer on low speed, add dry ingredients and hot water. Mix together.
4. Divide batter between prepared pans and bake for 20–25 minutes, or until wooden pick inserted in center comes out almost clean. Cool brownies for 10 minutes. Run a sharp knife around edges of pan to loosen brownies. Turn out onto wire rack.
5. To assemble, place one brownie layer on serving plate. Top with ⅔ of cherry pie filling. Place second brownie layer on top of cherry pie filling. Top with remaining cherry pie filling. Serve with whipped topping and a scant 1 tablespoon of chocolate syrup.

Nutrition Information (per serving)

Calories 300 • Fat 5g • Protein 3g • Carbohydrates 67g • Cholesterol 25mg • Sodium 180mg • Fiber 2g

*__Black Forest Brownie Torte Without Eggs:__ Omit egg and add 1 tablespoon Ener-G egg replacer powder. Increase hot water or coffee by ½ cup. Bake as directed.

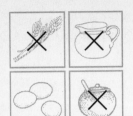

CARROT CAKE

Serves 16

Rich, dense, and utterly decadent. This is one of my all-time, most favorite recipes.

2½ cups Flour Blend (page 276)

2 teaspoons baking soda

2 teaspoons ground cinnamon

1½ teaspoons xanthan gum

1 teaspoon salt

½ teaspoon ground ginger

4 large eggs

1 cup packed light brown sugar
or maple sugar

1 cup granulated sugar or fructose
powder

⅓ cup canola oil

1 cup plain nonfat yogurt, or ¾ cup
2% milk (cow, rice, or soy)

1 teaspoon vanilla extract

3 cups shredded carrots

1½ cups crushed pineapple, drained

1 cup shredded coconut

1 cup chopped walnuts

CREAM CHEESE FROSTING (OPTIONAL)

⅓ cup softened low-fat cream cheese
or soft silken tofu

2 cups powdered sugar or fructose
powder

2 tablespoons 2% milk (cow, rice,
or soy)

1 teaspoon vanilla extract

1. Preheat oven to 350°F. Grease 10-cup Bundt cake pan. Combine dry ingredients (flour to ginger) in bowl and set aside.

2. In large mixer bowl, beat eggs, sugars, oil, yogurt, and vanilla with electric mixer until smooth. Add flour mixture slowly on low speed, then increase speed to medium and beat until smooth. With large spatula, stir in carrots, pineapple, coconut, and nuts. Pour batter into prepared pan.

3. Bake for 45–50 minutes, or until wooden pick inserted in center of cake comes out clean. Cool on wire rack. Remove cake from pan.

4. To make cream cheese frosting, combine all frosting ingredients in bowl. Beat until smooth. Spread over cake, if desired.

Nutrition Information (per slice with frosting)
Calories 400 • Fat 9g • Protein 5g • Carbohydrates 77g • Cholesterol 47mg • Sodium 366mg • Fiber 1.5g

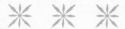

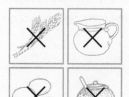

CARAMELIZED PEAR TORTE

Serves 12

This is a fabulous winter dessert. It is best made in a cast-iron skillet so you don't have to pour the caramel into another dish.

¾ cup packed light brown sugar or maple sugar

2 tablespoons water

3 firm ripe pears

⅓ cup butter or margarine, at room temperature, or canola oil

1 cup granulated sugar or fructose powder

2 large eggs*

1 tablespoon grated lemon zest

1½ cups Flour Blend (page 276)

1 teaspoon xanthan gum

½ teaspoon baking powder

½ teaspoon baking soda

¼ teaspoon salt

½ cup buttermilk, or 2 teaspoons vinegar or lemon juice and enough nondairy milk to equal ½ cup

1 teaspoon vanilla extract

1. Preheat oven to 350°F. In a greased 10-inch cast-iron skillet, combine sugar and water. Bring to simmer over low heat, swirling pan occasionally, until sugar dissolves. Cook another minute, gently swirling pan if sugar colors unevenly. Remove from heat. Cool for 10 minutes.
2. Wash and peel pears. Cut in half lengthwise, then in quarters. Remove core from each piece. Cut each quarter into 3 uniform wedges. Arrange pears in pinwheel design in caramel.

3. Using electric mixer and large mixer bowl, cream butter and sugar on medium speed until thoroughly blended. Mix in eggs and lemon zest on low speed until mixture is very smooth.

4. In medium bowl, sift the dry ingredients (flour through salt). In another medium bowl, combine buttermilk and vanilla.

5. On low speed, beat dry ingredients into butter mixture, alternating with buttermilk. Mix well and pour batter over pears.

6. Bake for 30–35 minutes, or until wooden pick inserted in center comes out clean. Cool for 5 minutes. Loosen edges with knife. Using hot mitts, invert torte onto serving plate. Remove skillet. Cool to room temperature.

Nutrition Information (per serving)
Calories 285 • Fat 7g • Protein 3g • Carbohydrates 57g • Cholesterol 44mg • Sodium 150mg • Fiber 1g

*__Caramelized Pear Torte Without Eggs:__ Use Basic Cake Without Eggs on page 172.

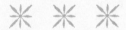

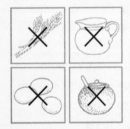

CHOCOLATE CHERRY CAKE

Serves 12

If you like the combination of chocolate and cherries, then try this recipe. For variety, try the sweeter Bing cherries. This produces a heavy, dense cake—especially if you use the tofu.

1¼ cups Flour Blend (page 276)
½ cup unsweetened cocoa powder (not Dutch process)
1 teaspoon xanthan gum

1 teaspoon baking soda
¾ teaspoon salt
¾ cup packed light brown sugar or maple sugar

2 teaspoons vanilla extract

1 teaspoon almond extract

½ cup 2% milk (cow, rice, or soy)

½ cup (1 stick) butter or margarine, at room temperature, or ⅓ cup canola oil

1 large egg, or ¼ cup soft silken tofu

½ cup warm coffee or water (110°F)

1 can (16 ounces) tart cherries, drained

1. Preheat oven to 350°F. Grease 9-inch round or 9-inch square nonstick baking pan. In mixer bowl, combine flours, cocoa, xanthan gum, baking soda, and salt.

2. In food processor, process sugar, vanilla and almond extracts, milk, butter, and egg until smooth. Add warm coffee and blend until very smooth. Add flour mixture and mix at low speed until smooth. Add cherries; pulse until incorporated.

3. Spoon batter into prepared pan and bake for 25–30 minutes, or until top is firm and wooden pick inserted in center comes out clean. Remove from oven. Cool for 5 minutes before removing cake from pan.

Nutrition Information (per serving)
Calories 225 • Fat 9g • Protein 3g • Carbohydrates 37g • Cholesterol 36mg • Sodium 330mg • Fiber 2g

Variations

Cupcakes: Bake 12 cupcakes for 20–25 minutes, or until wooden pick inserted in center comes out clean.

Layer Cake: Bake in two greased 9-inch round nonstick baking pans for 30–35 minutes, or two 8-inch round nonstick cake baking pans for 25–30 minutes, or until wooden pick inserted in center comes out clean. Also, first line pan(s) with waxed paper or parchment paper and grease again for easier cake removal. Frost with desired frosting. (See frosting section, pages 197–204.) Serves 12.

CHOCOLATE MACAROON TUNNEL CAKE

Serves 12

This cake combines two of the most wonderful flavors on earth—chocolate and coconut. Finish off with your favorite frosting and a little toasted coconut sprinkled on top.

2¼ cups Flour Blend (page 276)
1½ teaspoons xanthan gum
1½ teaspoons baking soda
1 teaspoon salt
1¼ cups granulated sugar or
    fructose powder
2 large eggs*
½ cup canola oil
1 tablespoon vanilla extract
1 teaspoon coconut extract

¾ cup buttermilk, or 1 tablespoon
    vinegar or lemon juice with
    enough nondairy milk to equal
    ¾ cup
¾ cup warm water (110°F)
½ cup shredded coconut
2 teaspoons coconut extract
⅔ cup unsweetened cocoa powder
    (not Dutch process)

1. Preheat oven to 350°F. Grease a 10-inch nonstick Bundt cake pan. Combine flours, xanthan gum, baking soda, and salt in small bowl and set aside.
2. In large mixer bowl, blend sugar or fructose powder, eggs, oil, and vanilla and coconut extracts with electric mixer until thoroughly blended. Add dry ingredients and buttermilk alternately, beginning and ending with dry ingredients. Add warm water and mix until thoroughly blended. Remove ⅔ cup batter and combine with coconut and coconut extract.
3. To remaining batter, beat in cocoa with electric mixer until thoroughly blended. Pour half of chocolate batter into pan, spreading evenly. Carefully spoon coconut batter over center of chocolate batter to form uniform ring, making sure not to let coconut batter touch sides of pan.
4. Carefully pour remaining chocolate batter into prepared pan, taking care not to disturb coconut ring. Gently spread chocolate batter to edges of pan as evenly as possible.
5. Bake for 40–45 minutes, or until wooden pick inserted in center comes out clean.

Nutrition Information (per serving)

Calories 350 • Fat 12g • Protein 4g • Carbohydrates 62g • Cholesterol 31mg • Sodium 362mg • Fiber 2g

*Chocolate Macaroon Tunnel Cake Without Eggs: Prepare Basic Chocolate Cake Without Eggs (page 175) and add coconut and coconut extract to ⅔ cup batter. Follow steps 3–5 of recipe above.

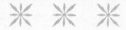

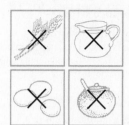

DOUBLE CHOCOLATE CHERRY TORTE

Serves 12

You can use tart red cherries or Bing cherries in this flavorful dessert.

FILLING

¼ cup 2% milk (cow, rice, or soy)

½ cup gluten-free, dairy-free chocolate chips

CAKE

1 can (16 ounces) cherries with ¼ cup juice reserved for sauce

1 cup packed light brown sugar or maple sugar

⅔ cup Flour Blend (page 276)

½ cup unsweetened cocoa powder (not Dutch process)

1 teaspoon xanthan gum

1 teaspoon baking soda

¾ teaspoon salt

½ teaspoon baking powder

⅓ cup canola oil

2 teaspoons vanilla extract

1 teaspoon almond extract

2 large eggs, or ½ cup soft silken tofu

½ cup sliced almonds

2 teaspoons water

SAUCE

¼ cup reserved cherry juice

¼ cup unsweetened cocoa powder (not Dutch process)

2 tablespoons canola oil

⅓ cup honey or agave nectar

1. Combine milk and chocolate chips in a small saucepan over low heat and stir until smooth. Set aside.
2. Preheat oven to 325°F. In blender, puree cherries with ¼ cup of their juice and set aside. Grease 8-inch nonstick springform pan.
3. In large mixer bowl, combine sugar, flours, cocoa, xanthan gum, baking soda, salt, and baking powder with electric mixer on low speed. Blend in oil, vanilla, and almond extract. Set aside ½ cup of mixture, which will be dry and crumbly.
4. To remaining mixture, mix in pureed cherries and eggs or tofu. Spread batter in prepared pan; top with reserved filling. Stir nuts and water into ½ cup reserved dry cake mixture and sprinkle over filling.
5. Bake for 50 minutes, or until top of cake is firm. Cool in pan on wire rack for 10 minutes. Remove from pan. Cool.
6. To prepare sauce, combine ingredients in blender and process until completely smooth. Drizzle over each serving.

Nutrition Information (per serving)
Calories 370 • Fat 15g • Protein 5g • Carbohydrates 45g • Cholesterol 30mg • Sodium 275mg • Fiber 3g

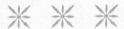

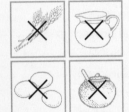

PINEAPPLE UPSIDE-DOWN CAKE

Serves 12

Serve this all-American favorite on a big, colorful platter for a pretty effect.

> ½ cup packed light brown sugar or maple sugar
> 1 can (14.5–16 ounces) pineapple rings in juice, drained
> 7 maraschino cherries or fresh raspberries
> 1 recipe Basic Cake (page 171) or Basic Cake
>   Without Eggs (page 172)

1. Preheat oven to 350°F.
2. Grease 10-inch pie plate or skillet (or special pan designed for upside-down cake). Sprinkle brown sugar evenly over bottom of pan. Arrange pineapple slices with cherry (or raspberry) in center of each circle. Pour cake batter evenly on top.
3. Bake for 40–45 minutes, or until top springs back when touched. Cool for 5 minutes, then invert onto serving plate.

Nutrition Information (per serving with eggs)

Calories 450 • Fat 8g • Protein 3g • Carbohydrates 94g • Cholesterol 31 mg • Sodium 206mg • Fiber 2g

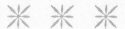

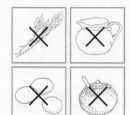

CHOCOLATE FUDGE TORTE

Serves 12

You would never guess that this fabulous torte has no eggs, and you'll love the texture.

FILLING
½ cup gluten-free, dairy-free chocolate chips
¼ cup 2% milk (cow, rice, or soy)

CAKE
1 cup Flour Blend (page 276)
½ cup unsweetened cocoa powder (not Dutch process)
½ teaspoon xanthan gum
¾ teaspoon baking soda
½ teaspoon baking powder
¾ teaspoon salt

2 teaspoons ground cinnamon
1 cup packed light brown sugar or maple sugar
1 teaspoon egg replacer powder
⅓ cup canola oil
2 teaspoons vanilla extract
1 can (16 ounces) canned pears, drained
2 eggs, or ⅓ cup hot coffee (115°F)
½ cup chopped nuts of choice (optional)
2 teaspoons water

1. Combine chocolate chips and milk in a small saucepan over low heat (or melt in microwave) and stir until smooth. Set aside.

2. Preheat oven to 325°F. Grease 8-inch nonstick springform pan.

3. In large mixer bowl, mix flours, cocoa, xanthan gum, baking soda, baking powder, salt, cinnamon, brown sugar, and egg replacer together with oil and vanilla to make dry, crumbly mixture. Remove and reserve ½ cup. In blender or food processor, puree drained pears. (Discard juice.)

4. In large mixer bowl, thoroughly mix dry cake mixture, pureed pears, and eggs or hot coffee with electric mixer. Spread batter into prepared pan. Spoon reserved chocolate filling onto top of batter. Stir nuts (if using) and water into remaining ½ cup dry cake mixture and sprinkle over filling.

5. Bake for 50 minutes, or until top is firm. Cool on wire rack for 10 minutes, then remove from pan. Cool completely. Serve with Chocolate Fudge Sauce (page 196) or Chocolate Frosting (page 199).

Nutrition Information (per serving)
Calories 270 • Fat 13g • Protein 3g • Carbohydrates 42g • Cholesterol 1mg • Sodium 237mg • Fiber 3.5g

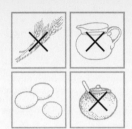

FLOURLESS CHOCOLATE CAKE

Serves 8

This is one of my old standby recipes—the one I make when I want a sure winner. If you're in a huge hurry, just add the whole eggs without beating the egg whites separately. The cake will be heavier, but still delicious. Since this cake relies on eggs for leavening, it isn't egg free.

2 cups walnut halves
1 cup packed light brown sugar
   or maple sugar
½ cup light olive oil
½ cup Dutch-process cocoa powder

1 teaspoon vanilla extract
⅛ teaspoon salt
5 large eggs, separated
Frosting, melted chocolate, or
   powdered sugar, to top (optional)

1. Preheat oven to 350°F. Grease 8- or 9-inch nonstick springform pan.
2. Grind nuts in food processor to cornmeal-like texture. Add sugar, oil, cocoa, vanilla, salt, and egg yolks and blend until thoroughly mixed.
3. In separate large mixer bowl with clean beaters, beat egg whites with electric mixer until soft peaks form.
4. Gently fold cocoa mixture into beaten egg whites, adding ¼ of the mixture at a time.
5. Pour batter into prepared pan. Bake for 40–45 minutes, or until wooden pick inserted in center comes out clean. Cake rises as it bakes, then falls slightly as it cools. Cool for 15 minutes in pan on wire rack. Cut around edge to loosen cake from pan edges. Release pan sides. Slice into 8 pieces. Top with your favorite frosting, glaze with melted chocolate, or dust with powdered sugar.

Nutrition Information (per serving)
Calories: 280 • Fat 21g • Protein 6g • Carbohydrates 21g • Sodium 75mg • Cholesterol 113mg • Fiber 1.5g

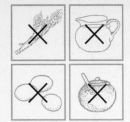

CHOCOLATE RASPBERRY CAKE

Serves 16

The raspberries in this cake make it exceptionally moist and lend a wonderful fruity note.

2½ cups Flour Blend (page 276)

2 cups packed light brown sugar or maple sugar

1 cup unsweetened cocoa powder (not Dutch process)

2½ teaspoons baking soda

2 teaspoons xanthan gum

1½ teaspoons salt

1 cup 2% milk (cow, rice, or soy)

1 cup (2 sticks) butter or margarine

2 large eggs*

2 teaspoons vanilla extract

¼ cup warm coffee or water (110°F)

1 cup thoroughly crushed raspberries

Raspberry Filling (page 202)

Chocolate Frosting (page 199)

½ cup raspberry jam, slightly warmed

Fresh flowers and fresh raspberries, for garnish

1. Preheat oven to 350°F. Grease two 9-inch round nonstick baking pans. Line with waxed paper and grease again.
2. Blend all ingredients except coffee and raspberries in large mixer bowl with electric mixer. Add coffee and raspberries and mix until thoroughly blended. Pour into prepared pans. Bake for 35–40 minutes, or until wooden pick inserted in center comes out clean. Cool for 5 minutes. Turn cakes out of pans onto wire rack and remove paper. Cool thoroughly.
3. Slice each layer in half horizontally. Brush away excess crumbs.
4. Have raspberry filling and chocolate frosting ready. To assemble, place first layer on cake stand. Brush with thin layer of raspberry jam. Spread thin layer of raspberry filling on top of jam. Repeat with remaining cake layers. Chill cake for 30 minutes.
5. Frost with chocolate frosting. Decorate with fresh flowers and fresh raspberries sprinkled around cake.

Nutrition Information (per serving)

Calories 445 • Fat 18g • Protein 5g • Carbohydrates 73g • Cholesterol 73mg • Sodium 660mg • Fiber 4g

*Chocolate Raspberry Cake Without Eggs: Use Basic Chocolate Cake Without Eggs (page 175). Double the recipe, but use 2½ teaspoons baking powder. Add raspberries with other liquid ingredients.

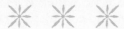

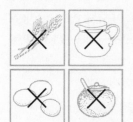

COCONUT CAKE

Serves 12

Coconut fans will love this cake because it is loaded with coconut—in the cake, in the frosting, and sprinkled on top for a decorative touch.

⅓ cup butter or margarine, at room
   temperature

1 cup granulated sugar or fructose
   powder

2 large eggs*

1½ cups Flour Blend (page 276)

1 teaspoon xanthan gum

½ teaspoon baking powder

½ teaspoon baking soda

¼ teaspoon salt

¼ cup shredded coconut

¾ cup buttermilk, or 1 tablespoon
   vinegar or lemon juice with
   enough nondairy milk to equal
   ¾ cup

1 teaspoon vanilla extract

1 teaspoon coconut extract

1 teaspoon almond extract

7-Minute White Frosting (page 204)
   or your favorite frosting

¼ cup shredded coconut

1 cup coconut flakes, lightly toasted

1. Preheat oven to 325°F. Grease two 8-inch round cake pans and line with waxed paper and grease again.
2. In large mixer bowl, cream butter and sugar with electric mixer on medium speed until light and fluffy. Mix in eggs.

3. In medium mixer bowl, sift together flour, xanthan gum, baking powder, baking soda, and salt.

4. In another medium mixer bowl, combine coconut, buttermilk, and extracts. On low speed, beat dry ingredients into butter mixture, alternating with buttermilk mixture. Spoon batter into prepared pans.

5. Bake for about 30 minutes, or until tops are golden brown and wooden pick inserted in center comes out clean. Let cakes cool in pans for 5 minutes, then remove from pans, remove parchment paper, and cool on wire rack.

6. Prepare white frosting of choice. To make coconut filling, stir ¼ cup shredded coconut into ½ cup frosting. Assemble cakes by placing layer on cake stand. Using a spatula, spread coconut filling on cake, working from the center of cake out to edges. Add second layer and frost top and edges of cake with a wide knife. Sprinkle toasted coconut flakes on cake.

Nutrition Information (per serving)

Calories 245 • Fat 7g • Protein 3g • Carbohydrates 44g • Cholesterol 44mg • Sodium 197mg • Fiber 0.5g

*Coconut Cake Without Eggs: Prepare Basic Cake Without Eggs (page 172) batter. Follow steps 4–6 of recipe above.

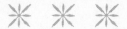

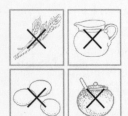

LEMON CAKE

Serves 16

Wonderfully lemony, this cake is a delightful choice for any occasion.

½ cup (1 stick) butter or margarine, or ⅓ cup canola oil	4 large eggs*
	½ cup grated lemon zest
2 cups granulated sugar or fructose powder	3 cups Flour Blend (page 276)
	1½ teaspoons xanthan gum

½ teaspoon baking powder

½ teaspoon baking soda

½ teaspoon salt

1½ cups buttermilk, or 1 tablespoon vinegar or lemon juice with enough nondairy milk to equal 1½ cups

2 teaspoons vanilla extract

Orange marmalade

¼ cup grated lemon zest

7-Minute White Frosting (page 204) or white frosting of choice

Fresh mint leaves and edible flowers, for garnish

1. Preheat oven to 325°F. Grease two 9-inch round nonstick baking pans. Line with waxed paper and grease again.
2. In large mixer bowl, cream together butter and sugar with electric mixer on medium speed. Mix in eggs and lemon zest and set aside.
3. In medium mixer bowl, sift together flour, xanthan gum, baking powder, baking soda, and salt.
4. In another medium mixer bowl, combine buttermilk and vanilla. On low speed, beat dry ingredients into butter mixture, alternating with buttermilk. Spoon batter into prepared pans and smooth tops.
5. Bake for 30 minutes, or until tops are golden brown and wooden pick inserted in center comes out clean. Cool cakes in pans for 5 minutes. Remove from pans and cool on wire rack.
6. Slice layers in half horizontally. Place layer on cake stand; brush on thin glaze of marmalade. Repeat with remaining layer. Chill.
7. Stir lemon zest into white frosting. Frost cake with wide spatula using dips and swirls to create decorative effect. Garnish with mint leaves and flowers.

Nutrition Information (per serving)

Calories 500 • Fat 10g • Protein 5g • Carbohydrates 103g • Cholesterol 82mg • Sodium 299mg • Fiber 1g

*Lemon Cake Without Eggs:** Use Basic Cake Without Eggs (page 172). Double the recipe, but use 2½ teaspoons baking powder.

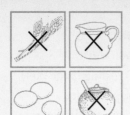

SPICE CAKE

Serves 16

The aroma of this cake baking in the oven will tantalize your taste buds. See the egg-free version on page 193.

3 cups Flour Blend (page 276)

1½ teaspoons xanthan gum

1 teaspoon baking soda

1 teaspoon salt

1½ tablespoons ground ginger

3 teaspoons ground cinnamon

¾ teaspoon ground nutmeg

¼ teaspoon ground cloves

2¼ cups 2% milk (cow, rice, or soy)

2¼ cups packed light brown sugar or maple sugar

½ cup canola oil

½ cup molasses or maple syrup

1½ teaspoons vanilla extract

3 large eggs

7-Minute White Frosting (page 204) or white frosting of choice

1 tablespoon instant coffee powder

1 tablespoon hot water

Shaved chocolate, Dutch-process cocoa powder, or chopped nuts of choice, for garnish (optional)

1. Preheat oven to 325°F. Grease two 8- or 9-inch round nonstick baking pans. Line bottoms with waxed paper and grease again.
2. In large mixer bowl, sift together flours, xanthan gum, baking soda, salt, and spices.
3. Bring milk and sugar to boiling in heavy saucepan over medium heat. Remove from heat. Add oil, molasses, and vanilla.
4. Add milk mixture to flour mixture and mix until thoroughly blended. Add eggs and mix until blended. Pour batter into prepared pans.
5. Bake for 35–40 minutes, or until wooden pick inserted in center comes out clean. Cool cakes in pans for 5 minutes. Invert cakes onto plate or wire rack to finish cooling. Remove paper.
6. Slice each layer in half horizontally. Brush excess crumbs away.
7. Prepare frosting, adding instant coffee powder dissolved in hot water. Place one cake layer on serving plate. Spread thin layer of frosting on bottom half. Repeat with remaining layers. Frost sides and top with deep swirls in decorative manner. Garnish with shaved chocolate, cocoa powder, or chopped nuts, if desired.

Nutrition Information (per serving without garnishes)

Calories 470 • Fat 12g • Protein 5g • Carbohydrates 89g • Cholesterol 49mg • Sodium 440mg • Fiber 1g

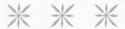

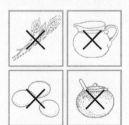

SPICE CAKE WITHOUT EGGS

Serves 16

For an interesting taste, try using brewed coffee as the liquid for the frosting.

2¾ cups Flour Blend (page 276)

1½ teaspoons xanthan gum

1½ teaspoons baking powder

1 teaspoon baking soda

1 teaspoon salt

1 tablespoon ground ginger

1 tablespoon ground cinnamon

½ teaspoon ground nutmeg

½ teaspoon ground cloves

1 cup packed light brown sugar or maple sugar

1½ cups boiling water, divided

¾ cup soft silken tofu

¾ cup molasses or maple syrup

1½ teaspoons vanilla extract

½ cup canola oil

7-Minute White Frosting (page 204) or frosting of choice

1 tablespoon instant coffee powder

1 tablespoon hot water

Shaved chocolate, Dutch-process cocoa powder, or chopped nuts of choice, for garnish (optional)

1. Preheat oven to 325°F. Grease two 8- or 9-inch round nonstick cake pans. Line with waxed paper and grease again.

2. In large mixer bowl, sift flours, xanthum gum, baking powder, baking soda, salt, and spices. Dissolve sugar in 1 cup boiling water (reserve remaining water).

3. In large mixer bowl, blend tofu, dissolved sugar mixture, molasses, and vanilla with electric mixer until very smooth. Add flour mixture and mix just until combined.

Add remaining boiling water and oil. Blend again, scraping sides of bowl with spatula. Batter will be somewhat thick. Pour batter into prepared pans.

4. Bake for 30–35 minutes, or until wooden pick inserted in center comes out clean. Remove from oven. Cool for 10 minutes. Remove from pans, remove paper, and cool on wire rack.

5. Prepare frosting of choice, adding instant coffee powder dissolved in hot water. Place first layer on serving plate and spread with ½ cup frosting. Add top layer and frost sides and top with spatula using deep, decorative swirls. Garnish with shaved chocolate, cocoa powder, or chopped nuts, if desired.

Nutrition Information (per serving without garnishes)
Calories 385 • Fat 11g • Protein 3g • Carbohydrates 73g • Cholesterol 0mg • Sodium 343mg • Fiber 1g

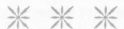

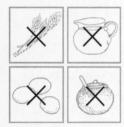

WHITE CAKE WITH FRUIT FILLING

Serves 12

This cake is especially pretty with the colorful raspberry and apricot layers. It is a small cake, but you can always bake several of them if you are entertaining many guests.

⅓ cup butter or margarine, at room temperature, or ¼ cup canola oil
1 cup granulated sugar or fructose powder
3 large egg whites*
1½ cups Flour Blend (page 276)
1 teaspoon xanthan gum

½ teaspoon baking powder
½ teaspoon baking soda
¼ teaspoon salt
¾ cup buttermilk, or 2 teaspoons vinegar or lemon juice with enough nondairy milk to equal ¾ cup

1 teaspoon vanilla extract
1 teaspoon almond extract
Raspberry Filling (page 202)
1 cup apricot preserves

7-Minute White Frosting (page 204)
or frosting of choice
Fresh raspberries, dried apricot slivers,
or fresh mint, for garnish

1. Preheat oven to 325°F. Grease three 8-inch round nonstick cake pans. Line with waxed paper and grease again.
2. In large mixer bowl, cream butter and sugar with electric mixer on medium speed until blended. Mix in egg whites.
3. In medium mixer bowl, sift together flours, xanthan gum, baking powder, baking soda, and salt.
4. In another medium mixer bowl, combine buttermilk, and vanilla and almond extracts. On low speed, beat dry ingredients into butter mixture, alternating with buttermilk. Spoon batter into prepared pans.
5. Bake for 25–30 minutes, until tops are golden brown and wooden pick inserted in center comes out clean. Cool cakes in pans for 5 minutes. Remove cakes from pans, remove paper, and cool on wire rack.
6. Place one layer on plate. Spread raspberry filling with spatula, working from center to edges. Repeat process for next tier, using apricot preserves. Place third tier on top. Refrigerate cake for 1 hour.
7. Frost top layer and edges of cake with white frosting, using a wide knife, making swirls and dips for a decorative effect. Garnish with raspberries, apricots, or mint.

Nutrition Information (per serving)
Calories 285 • Fat 6g • Protein 3g • Carbohydrates 56g • Cholesterol 14mg • Sodium 196mg • Fiber 1.5g

*White Cake Without Eggs: Use Basic Cake Without Eggs (page 172). Fill, frost, and decorate as directed.

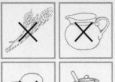
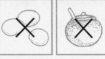

CHOCOLATE FUDGE SAUCE

Serves 16

Rich and high on the chocolate flavor scale, this sauce is great on cake, fruit, or ice cream. This sauce is doubly rich when made with whole milk or cream, but it also works well with 2% milk.

1 cup packed light brown sugar or
   maple sugar
¼ cup honey or agave nectar
⅓ cup canola oil

½ cup 2% milk (cow, rice, or soy)
2 teaspoons vanilla extract
¼ cup gluten-free, dairy-free
   chocolate chips

Combine sugar, honey, and oil in small, heavy pan over medium heat. Bring to boiling, then simmer gently over very low heat for 5 minutes without stirring. Remove from heat and stir in milk, vanilla, and chocolate chips until smooth.

Nutrition Information (per serving)
Calories 110 • Fat 5g • Protein 1g • Carbohydrates 15g • Cholesterol 1g • Sodium 8mg •
   Fiber 0mg

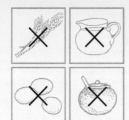

CHOCOLATE ESPRESSO GANACHE

Frosts the top of one 9-inch double-layer cake to serve 12

You've seen the lovely, shiny finish on gourmet cakes. Make your own with this easy recipe. It will work better with whole milk or cream, but I make it here with 2% milk.

> 12 ounces gluten-free, dairy-free bittersweet
>   or semisweet chocolate chips
> ½ cup 2% milk (cow, rice, or soy)
> 1 tablespoon butter, margarine, or canola oil
> 1 tablespoon espresso powder

1. Place chocolate chips in heatproof bowl. Heat milk and butter in small saucepan until bubbles appear around edge. Remove from heat and add espresso, stirring to dissolve.
2. Pour hot milk over chocolate. Let stand 1 minute, then stir until melted and smooth. Let stand at room temperature for 10 minutes before using. Pour over cake or dessert while lukewarm and spread on top with spatula. Serve within 30 minutes before ganache hardens and loses its sheen.

Nutrition Information (per serving)
Calories 150 • Fat 8g • Protein 2g • Carbohydrates 20g • Cholesterol 3mg • Sodium 13mg •
   Fiber 0.5g

Variation
For pure chocolate ganache, leave out the espresso.

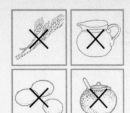

CHOCOLATE SYRUP

Serves 8

Use this syrup whenever the recipe calls for chocolate syrup. It is great drizzled on cakes when you don't want to use frosting, and it's a little thinner than the Chocolate Fudge Sauce on page 196.

> 3 tablespoons 2% milk (cow, rice, or soy)
> 2 tablespoons butter or margarine
> ¼ cup unsweetened cocoa powder (not Dutch process)
> 5 tablespoons honey or agave nectar

Combine all ingredients in blender and process until completely smooth. Refrigerate, covered.

Nutrition Information (per serving)
Calories 65 • Fat 3g • Protein 1g • Carbohydrates 11g • Cholesterol 1mg • Sodium 5mg • Fiber 1g

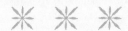

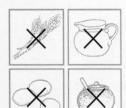

CHOCOLATE CHIP FROSTING

Frosts one double-layer cake to serve 12

A very simple frosting that's sure to please *everyone*.

> 2 cups gluten-free, dairy-free chocolate chips
> ¼ cup honey or agave nectar
> ¼ cup 2% milk (cow, rice, or soy)

1 tablespoon butter or margarine or nut butter (almond or cashew)
1 teaspoon vanilla extract

Place all ingredients in glass bowl and microwave on Medium power for 2 minutes, stopping and stirring after a minute. If you prefer smooth frosting, process in food processor until very, very smooth, adding additional milk to reach spreading consistency. Otherwise, use frosting immediately or it will begin to harden.

Nutrition Information (per serving)
Calories 165 • Fat 9g • Protein 1g • Carbohydrates 22g • Cholesterol 3mg • Sodium 6mg • Fiber 2g

✳ ✳ ✳

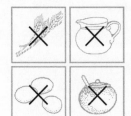

CHOCOLATE FROSTING

Frosts one 9-inch single-layer cake to serve 12

Another yummy chocolate frosting!

⅔ cup Chocolate Syrup (page 198)
1 tablespoon arrowroot powder
¼ cup rice milk

1. Place chocolate syrup in small, heavy saucepan. Dissolve arrowroot powder in milk, then stir mixture into chocolate syrup.
2. Heat mixture over low-medium setting, about 8–10 minutes, until it starts to thicken, stirring occasionally. Remove from heat and cool slightly. Mixture will thicken as it cools.
3. Frost a single-layer cake to serve 12, or 12 cupcakes. For larger cakes, double or triple the recipe. If frosting thickens too much, stir in 1 tablespoon of milk at a time to reach desired consistency.

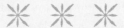

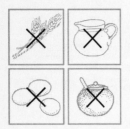

CHOCOLATE TOFU FROSTING

Frosts one double-layer cake to serve 12

This frosting has a rich, bold chocolate flavor with a creamy texture.

- ⅓ cup extra-firm silken tofu
- 2 cups pure maple syrup
- 2 cups unsweetened cocoa powder (not Dutch process)
- 1 tablespoon vanilla extract

Blend tofu with maple syrup in food processor or blender until completely smooth. Add cocoa and vanilla and blend until very, very smooth. Refrigerate frosting for 15 minutes before using.

Nutrition Information (per serving)

Calories 180 • Fat 2g • Protein 3g • Carbohydrates 44g • Cholesterol 0mg • Sodium 8mg • Fiber 5g

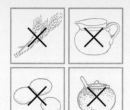

VANILLA FROSTING

Frosts one single-layer cake to serve 12

Use this frosting as a lower-sugar alternative to a traditional powdered-sugar frosting. Add almond or coconut extract for additional flavor.

1 package (12 ounces) extra-firm silken tofu

¼ cup granulated sugar or fructose powder

1 teaspoon fresh lemon juice

1 teaspoon butter or margarine

1 teaspoon vanilla extract

1 teaspoon butter-flavored extract

¼ teaspoon salt

¼ teaspoon xanthan gum

Drain tofu thoroughly in a mesh sieve for at least 2 hours. Discard liquid. Combine all ingredients in food processor and process mixture until very smooth, scraping down sides with spatula. Use immediately.

Nutrition Information (per serving)
Calories 35 • Fat 1g • Protein 1g • Carbohydrates 4g • Cholesterol 0mg • Sodium 50mg • Fiber 0g

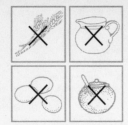

RASPBERRY FILLING

Fills one layer in two-layer cake recipe to serve 12

This is a lovely filling for a white or chocolate layer cake. Double the recipe if you want to fill and top a double-layer cake.

> 2 cups fresh raspberries
> ½ cup granulated sugar or fructose powder
> 2 tablespoons cornstarch
> 1 teaspoon vanilla extract

1. Mash fresh raspberries in small bowl until thoroughly crushed. Press mixture through sieve and discard seeds. Place crushed raspberries and sugar in small saucepan and whisk in cornstarch.
2. Place pan over medium heat, stirring until mixture thickens. Cook and stir 2 minutes more. Remove from heat and stir in vanilla. Transfer filling to small bowl, cover, and refrigerate for at least 2 hours.

Nutrition Information (per serving)
Calories 45 • Fat 0.5g • Protein 1g • Carbohydrates 11g • Cholesterol 0mg • Sodium 1mg • Fiber 1g

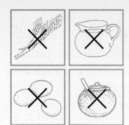

SOY~BASED
WHIPPED TOPPING

Makes ½ cup (Serves 4)

Tofu makes this topping smooth and creamy. Use it like any dairy whipped topping.

    ½ cup soft silken tofu
    2 tablespoons honey or agave nectar
    ½ teaspoon vanilla extract
    ¼ teaspoon butter-flavored extract
    ⅛ teaspoon salt

Combine all ingredients in blender or mini-food processor and process until very smooth. Refrigerate until ready to use.

Nutrition Information (per serving)
Calories 45 • Fat 1g • Protein 2g • Carbohydrates 8g • Cholesterol 0mg • Sodium 75mg • Fiber 0g

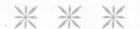

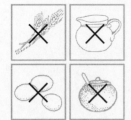

NUT~BASED
WHIPPED TOPPING

Makes 1 cup (Serves 8)

    ¾ cup raw cashews or almonds
    ¼ cup honey or agave nectar
    2 teaspoons vanilla extract

    ½ teaspoon butter-flavored extract
    ¼ cup water
    ¼ teaspoon salt

1. Place nuts on baking sheet and toast in 350°F oven for 5–8 minutes, until lightly toasted but not browned. Grind nuts finely in blender.
2. Add honey, vanilla, butter extract, water, and salt. Process mixture again for about 5–8 minutes, until very smooth. Refrigerate until ready to use.

Nutrition Information (per serving)
Calories 110 • Fat 5g • Protein 2g • Carbohydrates 17g • Cholesterol 0mg • Sodium 118mg • Fiber 0.5g

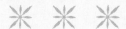

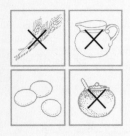

7-MINUTE WHITE FROSTING

Frosts one double-layer cake to serve 12

This traditional frosting is usually off-limits for many people with food sensitivities because it contains eggs. However, for many of you it will be just fine, so use it if you can. If you require an egg-free frosting, see page 201.

> 3 large egg whites
> 1¼ cups granulated sugar or fructose powder
> ¼ teaspoon cream of tartar
> 3 tablespoons cold water
> 1 teaspoon vanilla extract

Combine all ingredients in double boiler over boiling water. Beat with handheld electric mixer for 5–7 minutes, until glossy and mixture reaches desired spreading consistency. Use immediately.

Nutrition Information (per serving)
Calories 100 • Fat 0g • Protein 1g • Carbohydrates 25g • Cholesterol 0mg • Sodium 17mg • Fiber 0g

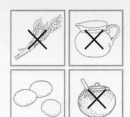

GINGERBREAD

Serves 12

You'll love the smell of this gingerbread, dark and deeply aromatic, wafting through your kitchen as it bakes.

GINGERBREAD

¼ cup canola oil

½ cup packed light brown sugar*

1 large egg

½ cup molasses

1 teaspoon vanilla extract

1½ cups Flour Blend (page 276)

1 teaspoon xanthan gum

1 teaspoon baking soda

1½ teaspoons ground ginger

¾ teaspoon ground cinnamon

½ teaspoon ground cloves

½ teaspoon salt

½ cup buttermilk, or 1 teaspoon
    vinegar or lemon juice and enough
    milk (cow, rice, or soy) to equal
    ½ cup

LEMON SAUCE

¼ cup granulated sugar or fructose
   powder

1 tablespoon cornstarch

⅛ teaspoon salt

½ cup water

2 teaspoons grated lemon zest

1 tablespoon fresh lemon juice

1 teaspoon canola oil

1. Preheat oven to 350°F. Grease 8- or 9-inch round or square nonstick baking pan. Cream oil and brown sugar with electric mixer in large mixer bowl. Add egg, molasses, and vanilla and beat well.

2. In large mixer bowl, mix flours with xanthan gum, baking soda, ginger, cinnamon, cloves, and salt. Add flours mixture alternately with buttermilk to creamed mixture. Pour into prepared pan.

3. Bake for 30 minutes, or until wooden pick inserted into center comes out clean. Cool in pan on wire rack.

4. To make lemon sauce, combine sugar, cornstarch, and salt in a small saucepan until blended. Gradually stir in water. Cook and stir over medium heat until mixture boils

and thickens. Stir in lemon zest, lemon juice, and oil. Cool slightly, then pour over each slice of gingerbread.

Nutrition Information (per serving)
Calories 235 • Fat 6g • Protein 2g • Carbohydrates 46g • Cholesterol 17mg • Sodium 244mg • Fiber 0.5g

*__Sugar Alternative:__ Use ⅓ cup pure maple syrup or honey in place of ½ cup brown sugar. Reduce buttermilk to ⅓ cup. Increase baking soda to 1⅛ teaspoons.

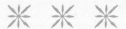

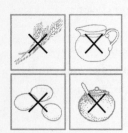

GINGERBREAD WITHOUT EGGS

Serves 12

Just as good as the egg version of gingerbread, this recipe is just a bit heavier in texture.

GINGERBREAD

1¾ cups Flour Blend (page 276)

1 teaspoon xanthan gum

1 teaspoon baking powder

¾ teaspoon baking soda

1 tablespoon ground ginger

1 teaspoon ground cinnamon

½ teaspoon ground cloves

¼ teaspoon ground nutmeg

¾ teaspoon salt

½ cup packed light brown sugar or maple sugar

1 cup boiling water

½ cup soft silken tofu

1 teaspoon vanilla extract

⅓ cup molasses or sorghum syrup

¼ cup canola oil

LEMON SAUCE

¼ cup granulated sugar or fructose powder

1 tablespoon cornstarch

⅛ teaspoon salt

½ cup water

2 teaspoons grated lemon zest

1 tablespoon fresh lemon juice

1 teaspoon canola oil

1. Preheat oven to 325°F. Coat 9-inch round nonstick cake pan with cooking spray. Measure flours, xanthan gum, baking powder, baking soda, ginger, cinnamon, cloves, nutmeg, and salt into small mixer bowl. Set aside.
2. In food processor, puree sugar, boiling water (reduce to ⅔ cup if using maple syrup), tofu, vanilla, and molasses until very, very smooth. Add oil and blend thoroughly. Add flour mixture and process until just blended. Batter will be somewhat thick. Pour into prepared pan.
3. Bake for 30–35 minutes, or until wooden pick inserted in center comes out clean. Remove from oven. Cool thoroughly before slicing.
4. To make lemon sauce, combine sugar, cornstarch, and salt in small saucepan until blended. Gradually stir in water. Cook and stir over medium heat until mixture boils and thickens. Stir in lemon zest, lemon juice, and oil. Cool slightly, then pour over each slice of gingerbread.

Nutrition Information (per serving)
Calories 250 • Fat 6g • Protein 2g • Carbohydrates 50g • Cholesterol 1mg • Sodium 280mg • Fiber 0.5g

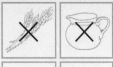

BASIC PIE CRUST

Makes 1 double crust or 2 single crusts (Serves 6)

1 cup Flour Blend (page 276)
¾ cup tapioca flour
½ cup sweet-rice flour
1 tablespoon + 1 teaspoon sugar
1 teaspoon xanthan gum
1 teaspoon guar gum
½ teaspoon salt

½ cup shortening
2 tablespoons butter or nondiet
  margarine
¼ cup 2% milk (cow, rice, or soy)
Rice flour, for dusting
½ large egg, for egg wash (optional)

FOR DOUBLE PIE CRUST:

1. Place flours, 1 tablespoon of sugar, gums, salt, shortening, and butter in food processor and process until well mixed. Add milk and blend until dough forms ball.

2. Flatten dough to 1-inch disk, wrap tightly, and chill for 1 hour so liquids are well distributed.

3. Massage dough between your hands until it is very pliable and no longer feels cold, making it easier to handle. Roll half of dough to 10-inch circle between two pieces of heavy-duty plastic wrap dusted with rice flour. Use damp paper towel between countertop and plastic wrap to anchor plastic wrap. (Keep remaining half wrapped tightly to avoid drying out.) Be sure to move rolling pin from center of dough to outer edge, moving around circle in clockwise fashion to assure uniform thickness.

4. Remove top plastic wrap and invert crust, centering it over pie plate. Remove remaining plastic wrap and press into place.

5. Fill crust with your choice of pie filling.

6. Roll remaining dough to 10-inch circle between floured plastic wrap. Invert and center on filled crust. Don't remove top plastic wrap until dough is centered. Shape decorative ridge around rim of pie plate. Prick crust several times with fork to allow steam to escape. Freeze pie for 15 minutes.

7. Brush with beaten egg, if desired, for shinier crust. Sprinkle with remaining teaspoon of sugar. Place on nonstick baking sheet. Bake according to instructions in your choice of pie recipe (usually until crust is golden brown).

Nutrition Information (per serving, crust only)

Calories 375 • Fat 22g • Protein 2g • Carbohydrates 44g • Sodium 203mg • Cholesterol 11mg •
Fiber 0.5g

FOR SINGLE PIE CRUST:

1. Place flours, 1 tablespoon of sugar, gums, salt, shortening, and butter in food processor and process until well mixed. Add milk and blend until dough forms ball.
2. Flatten dough to 1-inch disk, wrap tightly, and chill for 1 hour so liquids are well distributed.
3. Massage dough between your hands until it is very pliable and no longer feels cold, making it easier to handle. Roll half of dough to 10-inch circle between two pieces of heavy-duty plastic wrap dusted with rice flour. Use damp paper towel between countertop and plastic wrap to anchor plastic wrap. Be sure to move rolling pin from center of dough to outer edge, moving around circle in clockwise fashion to assure uniform thickness. Wrap and freeze remaining half for another pie.
4. Place crust in bottom of 9-inch nonstick pie plate. Shape a decorative edge around rim of pie. Freeze for 15 minutes.
5. To prepare a no-bake pie, brush the rim of pie crust with a beaten egg, if using, and prick bottom of crust with fork a few times so it bakes flat. Sprinkle with remaining teaspoon of sugar. Place pie plate on baking sheet and bake 10 minutes on lowest rack of preheated 375°F oven. Move to next higher rack of oven and bake another 10 minutes, or until pie crust rim is lightly browned. Remove from oven and cool thoroughly before adding no-bake filling. For a baked filling, follow the specific directions in your pie recipe.

Nutrition Information (per serving, crust only)

Calories 190 • Fat 11g • Protein 1g • Carbohydrates 24g • Sodium 100mg • Cholesterol 6mg •
Fiber 0g

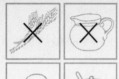
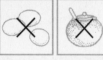

CRUMB PIE CRUST

Serves 6

This crust is a nice complement to smooth custard fillings that require no baking.

1 cup crushed egg-free cookie crumbs
(Vanilla Wafers on page 235;
Chocolate Wafers on page 229;
or "Graham" Crackers on
page 234)

¼ cup finely chopped nuts of choice
or pumpkin seeds, or 1¼ cups
crushed cookie crumbs
2 tablespoons canola oil
1 tablespoon brown sugar or maple sugar

Combine all ingredients in mixer bowl until well mixed and press into 9-inch microwave-safe pie plate. Cook for 2–3 minutes on High until firm. Fill crust with no-bake filling of your choice.

Nutrition Information (per serving)
Calories 200 • Fat 10g • Protein 1g • Carbohydrates 27g • Cholesterol 11mg • Sodium 185mg • Fiber 0.5g

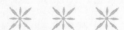

SPICY PEACH PIE

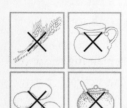

Serves 6

This pie is especially good when fresh peaches are in season. Be sure to measure the flour correctly: Gently whisk the flour to aerate it. Then lightly spoon it into the measuring cup without packing it down. Gently level the top with a straight knife. This is a double-crust pie.

1 Basic Pie Crust (page 208)
Rice flour, for dusting
4 cups sliced, peeled fresh peaches
(about 6 medium)
½ cup + 1 teaspoon granulated sugar
or fructose powder
¼ cup potato starch

2 teaspoons fresh lemon juice
½ teaspoon ground cinnamon
¼ teaspoon ground ginger
¼ teaspoon ground cardamom
¼ teaspoon salt
½ large egg, for egg wash (optional)

1. Prepare basic pie crust. Flatten dough to 1-inch disk, wrap tightly, and chill 1 hour so liquids are well distributed.
2. Massage the dough between your hands until it is very pliable and no longer feels cold, making it easier to handle. Roll half of the dough to a 10-inch circle between two pieces of heavy-duty plastic wrap dusted with rice flour. Use a damp paper towel between the countertop and plastic wrap to anchor the plastic wrap. (Keep remaining half wrapped tightly to avoid drying out.) Be sure to move the rolling pin from center of dough to the outer edge, moving around the circle in clockwise fashion to assure uniform thickness.
3. Remove top plastic wrap and invert crust, centering it over pie plate. Remove remaining plastic wrap and press into place.
4. In large mixer bowl, combine peaches, ½ cup sugar or fructose powder, potato starch, lemon juice, cinnamon, ginger, cardamom, and salt and toss until thoroughly blended. Drain away all but 2 tablespoons of juice.
5. Fill bottom pie crust with peach filling. Cover with top pie crust.
6. Roll remaining dough to 10-inch circle between floured plastic wrap. Invert and center on filled crust. Don't remove top plastic wrap until dough is centered. Shape decorative ridge around rim of pie plate. Prick crust several times with fork to allow steam to escape. Freeze for 15 minutes.
7. Brush with beaten egg, if desired, for shinier crust. Sprinkle with remaining teaspoon of sugar. Place on a nonstick baking sheet. Bake according to instructions in your choice of pie recipe (usually until crust is golden brown).
8. Preheat oven to 375°F. Bake for 15 minutes on lower rack. Move pie to center oven rack and bake for another 25–35 minutes, until crust is nicely browned. Cover loosely with foil if edges brown too much. Cool completely on wire rack before cutting.

Nutrition Information (per serving)
Calories 425 • Fat 17g • Protein 3g • Carbohydrates 72g • Sodium 235mg • Cholesterol 23mg • Fiber 2g

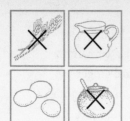

PUMPKIN PIE

Makes 1 pie (Serves 6)

This pie crust rolls out beautifully. With a little practice, you'll be a pro. Be sure to measure the flour correctly: Gently whisk the flour to aerate it. Then lightly spoon it into the measuring cup without packing it down. Gently level the top with a straight knife. This is a single-crust pie, and it contains eggs.

1 Basic Pie Crust (page 208)

Rice flour, for dusting

1 can (15 ounces) pure pumpkin (not pumpkin pie mix)

¾ cup granulated sugar or fructose powder

2 teaspoons pumpkin pie spice

1 teaspoon ground cinnamon

¾ teaspoon salt

2 eggs

1 cup 2% milk (cow, rice, or soy)

1. Prepare Basic Pie Crust. Flatten dough into two circular disks. Wrap both disks tightly, and freeze one for another use. Refrigerate remaining disk for 1 hour so liquids are well distributed throughout dough.
2. Massage chilled dough between hands until it is very pliable and no longer feels cold, making it easier to handle. Roll the dough to a 10-inch circle between two pieces of heavy-duty plastic wrap dusted with rice flour. Use damp paper towel on countertop to anchor plastic. Be sure to move the rolling pin from center of dough to the outer edge, moving around the circle in clockwise fashion to assure uniform thickness.
3. Remove top plastic wrap and invert crust, centering it over pie plate. Remove remaining plastic wrap and press into place. Flute edge of pie. Freeze 15 minutes.
4. Preheat oven to 425°F.
5. In large mixer bowl, beat pumpkin, sugar or fructose powder, spices, salt, eggs, and milk with electric mixer until smooth. Pour filling into pie crust.
6. Place pie on nonstick baking sheet. Bake for 15 minutes on lower rack. Move pie to center rack; reduce heat to 350°F and bake for 40–50 minutes, until knife inserted near center comes out clean. Cover edges of crust with foil if they brown too much. Cool 2 hours on wire rack. Serve immediately or refrigerate.

Nutrition Information (per serving)
Calories 295 • Fat 12g • Protein 4g • Carbohydrates 46g • Cholesterol 45mg • Sodium 224mg • Fiber 0.5g

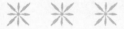

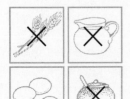

CLAFOUTI

Serves 6

Sort of like a big, thick pancake—but with fruit inside—this classic French dessert is easy to make and a great way to get more fruit into your diet. It is richer when made with whole milk, but I make it here with 2% milk. Since eggs are the leavening agent, it is not egg-free.

¼ cup Flour Blend (page 276)

¼ teaspoon salt

2 large eggs

⅓ cup 2% milk (cow, rice, or soy)

2 tablespoons honey or agave nectar

1 teaspoon vanilla extract

½ teaspoon grated lemon zest

2 tablespoons canola oil

3 cups peaches, cut into 1-inch cubes

2 tablespoons powdered sugar or fructose powder, pulverized in a small coffee grinder (optional)

1. Preheat oven to 375°F.
2. In blender, combine flours, salt, eggs, milk, honey, vanilla, lemon zest, and canola oil and whirl for 1 minute on high speed. (Or use immersion or handheld blender or wire whisk.) Batter will resemble pancake batter.
3. Grease 9-inch ovenproof skillet or pan or two small ovenproof skillets or pans. Pour in ¼ of batter, spreading over bottom of pan. Place skillet(s) in oven. Bake for 5–7 minutes, until batter resembles a cooked pancake.
4. Remove from heat. Put peaches on top of cooked batter. Top with remaining batter. Bake small skillets for 20–25 minutes, large skillet for 35–40 minutes, or until top is

puffy and golden brown. Remove from oven and dust with powdered sugar, if desired. Serve immediately.

Nutrition Information (per serving)

Calories 140 • Fat 7g • Protein 3g • Carbohydrates 18g • Cholesterol 63mg • Sodium 115mg • Fiber 2g

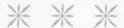

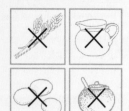

FRUIT TART

Serves 6

This is a nice summer dish when peaches are in season, but it works great with canned peaches, too.

   1 Single Pie Crust (page 209)
   7 canned peach halves, well drained
   ¾ cup peach preserves, melted

1. Preheat oven to 375°F. Press pie crust into 8-inch tart pan (similar to springform pan with removable rim). A regular pie pan will work if you don't have a tart pan, but the edges will be more slanted rather than straight up and down. Bake crust for 10 minutes.
2. Remove from oven. Place peach halves cut side down on crust. Brush tops of fruit and pie crust edges with melted preserves. Bake for 25–30 minutes, or until crust is nicely browned. Cool to room temperature before cutting.

Nutrition Information (per serving)

Calories 400 • Fat 12g • Protein 3g • Carbohydrates 77g • Cholesterol 14mg • Sodium 137mg • Fiber 4g

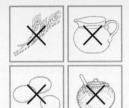

PEACH COBBLER

Serves 6

Substitute your own favorite fruit—perhaps cherries or blueberries—in this family favorite. Be sure to shake the buttermilk thoroughly before measuring.

1 cup Flour Blend (page 276)

½ cup granulated sugar or fructose powder

1 teaspoon baking powder

½ teaspoon xanthan gum

¼ teaspoon salt

¼ cup (½ stick) cold butter or margarine

⅓ cup buttermilk, or 1 teaspoon vinegar or lemon juice and enough nondairy milk (rice or soy) to equal ⅓ cup

1 large egg, or ¼ cup soft silken tofu

1 teaspoon grated lemon zest

1 teaspoon vanilla extract

3 cups sliced fresh peaches (about 3 large)

1 teaspoon sugar + ½ cup sugar or fructose powder

2 tablespoons potato starch

¼ teaspoon *each* cinnamon, nutmeg, and salt

1 teaspoon almond extract

1 teaspoon sugar

1. Preheat oven to 375°F. Grease 11x7-inch nonstick baking pan.
2. In mixer bowl, combine flours, sugar, baking powder, xanthan gum, and salt. Then cut in butter until mixture resembles peas.
3. In another mixer bowl, whisk together buttermilk, egg, lemon zest, and vanilla. Stir into dry ingredients until just mixed.
4. Prepare filling by combining peaches and 1 teaspoon sugar in large mixer bowl. Let stand for 30 minutes, then drain.
5. Combine ½ cup sugar, potato starch, cinnamon, nutmeg, and salt in small mixer bowl. Toss with drained peaches and almond extract. Place in prepared pan.
6. Drop cobbler topping onto filling by the tablespoonfuls. Sprinkle with sugar. Bake for 35–40 minutes on middle rack of oven, until nicely browned.

Nutrition Information (per serving)

Calories 400 • Fat 9g • Protein 3g • Carbohydrates 81g • Sodium 343mg • Cholesterol 31mg •
  Fiber 2g

Variation

Cherry Cobbler: Grease 8-inch square nonstick baking pan. Combine 2 cans (about 14.5 ounces each) drained tart red cherries, ¼ cup cherry juice, ⅔ cup sugar, 1 tablespoon quick-cooking tapioca, and 1 teaspoon almond extract in prepared pan. Let stand while preparing cobbler topping (steps 2 and 3). Add cobbler topping; bake as directed above.

Nutrition Information (per serving)

Calories 422 • Fat 9g • Protein 4g • Carbohydrates 85g • Sodium 346mg • Cholesterol 31mg •
  Fiber 1g

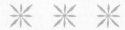

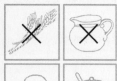
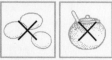

FLOWERPOT TREATS

Makes about 2 cups (Serves 4)

This is a delightful treat for children. They love to find the hidden treats inside the pudding. And, for some strange reason, children love the idea of eating dirt!

2 tablespoons unsweetened cocoa
  powder (not Dutch process)
½ cup packed light brown sugar or
  maple sugar

2 tablespoons cornstarch*
¼ teaspoon salt
2 cups 2% milk (cow, rice,* or soy)

1 ounce gluten-free, dairy-free
  bittersweet or semisweet
  chocolate pieces
1 teaspoon vanilla extract

4 small terra-cotta or plastic
  flowerpots
1 cup crushed Chocolate Wafers
  (page 229)

1. In medium-size, heavy saucepan, combine cocoa, sugar, cornstarch, and salt. Over medium heat, add milk. Whisk constantly, about 5–8 minutes, until mixture thickens.
2. Remove from heat and add chocolate and vanilla, stirring until chocolate melts. Chill thoroughly in refrigerator with a layer of plastic wrap pressed onto the top of the pudding to keep the top soft.
3. Assemble flowerpots (which have been cleaned thoroughly). Lay a piece of aluminum foil over hole in bottom.
4. Layer pudding and crushed chocolate wafers, ending with layer of crushed cookies. You can hide edible surprises inside, such as gluten-free gummy worms, fruit leather (cut in the shapes of worms), raisins, etc. Just make sure these items are safe for your diet.

Nutrition Information (per serving)
Calories 315 • Fat 6g • Protein 7g • Carbohydrates 62g • Cholesterol 4mg • Sodium 406mg • Fiber 2g

*If using rice milk, increase cornstarch to 3 tablespoons.

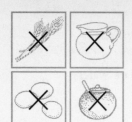

FROZEN TIRAMISU

Serves 12

This is a great way to use leftover cake. You can slice it in any shape you want as long as it is about 1 inch thick. The amount of ice cream is a matter of personal choice. Some people like lots of ice cream and just a little cake. The overall flavor of the dessert will vary depending on whether you use the espresso coffee or orange juice, but both versions are equally delicious. For maximum flavor, use both.

1 cup packed light brown sugar or maple sugar

1½ cups strong, freshly brewed espresso or fresh orange juice

1 recipe Basic Chocolate Cake (page 174) or Basic Chocolate Cake Without Eggs (page 175)

4 tablespoons finely ground espresso or grated orange zest, divided

2 pints Chocolate Cappuccino "Ice Cream" (page 240), divided

¼ cup Dutch-process cocoa powder

Grated chocolate or crushed gluten-free, dairy-free chocolate chips, for garnish

1. Dissolve sugar in espresso (or very strongly brewed coffee). Bring to boiling, reduce heat, and simmer for 1 minute to make espresso syrup. If using orange juice, follow same procedure but boil until mixture is reduced by ⅓, or about 1 cup. Remove from heat and let cool.

2. Slice cake into 1-inch-thick pieces with serrated knife. Place one layer in bottom of 9-inch square nonstick baking pan sprayed with cooking spray. Brush cake with espresso or orange syrup. Sprinkle 2 tablespoons of ground espresso or grated orange zest over cake. Spread half of softened ice cream over cake. Top with second layer of cake. Brush with remaining syrup.

3. Sprinkle with remaining 2 tablespoons ground espresso or orange zest. Top with remaining ice cream, creating decorative dips and swirls with back of spatula.

4. Return to freezer until completely frozen. At serving time, dust with Dutch cocoa and top with grated chocolate or crushed chocolate chips. Let stand at room temperature for a few minutes before serving.

Nutrition Information (per serving without garnishes)

Calories 400 • Fat 15g • Protein 6g • Carbohydrates 68g • Cholesterol 35mg • Sodium 412 mg • Fiber 3g

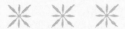

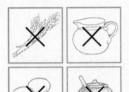

PANNA COTTA

Makes 2 cups (Serves 4)

Panna cotta is considered a rather trendy dessert these days, but it's actually just creamy gelatin with an Italian name. Of course, the original version is made with heavy cream. Try to use the heaviest, thickest nondairy milk you can find. Or perhaps stir in nondairy milk powder to the liquid milk you're using to boost its density.

1 tablespoon unflavored gelatin powder

2 cups 2% milk (cow, rice, or soy), divided

1 vanilla bean, or 1 teaspoon vanilla extract

¼ cup honey or agave nectar

1 teaspoon almond extract

⅛ teaspoon salt

1 cup fresh strawberries or raspberries

Fresh mint, for garnish

1. Sprinkle gelatin powder over ¼ cup of milk in small, heavy saucepan. Heat over very low heat for 3–5 minutes, until softened.
2. Meanwhile, in another saucepan, heat remaining milk and prepared vanilla bean (see Tip at end of recipe) until tiny bubbles form around edges of pan (do not boil). Remove from heat, remove vanilla bean, and stir in gelatin mixture, honey, almond extract, and salt until thoroughly mixed. (If you're not using vanilla bean, stir in vanilla extract now.)
3. Pour into 5-cup, decorative ring mold and refrigerate for 6 hours or overnight, until firm. (If you don't have such a mold, a Bundt cake pan will also work.)
4. Before unmolding the panna cotta, hull and slice strawberries.

5. To serve, dip the mold in lukewarm water and then dry bottom. Loosen edges with knife. Unmold onto serving platter. Spoon sliced strawberries in center of ring and garnish with fresh mint. Serve immediately.

Nutrition Information (per ½-cup serving)

Calories 130 • Fat 0.5g • Protein 6g • Carbohydrates 26g • Cholesterol 2mg • Sodium 140mg • Fiber 1g

Tip

Split vanilla bean lengthwise with a sharp knife. Scrape the seeds into milk and add scraped vanilla bean. After using, rinse scraped vanilla bean with water and place it in granulated sugar to add vanilla flavor.

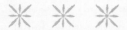

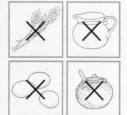

PEACH MELBA "ICE CREAM" PIE

Serves 10

For extra peach flavor and additional texture in the pie, stir in 1 cup of chopped peaches to the softened peach "ice cream" before spreading it in the pie plate. For variation, substitute a portion of the coconut—perhaps ¼ cup—with ground nuts such as pecans, walnuts, or hazelnuts.

CRUST

1½ cups shredded coconut
1 tablespoon sweet rice flour
¼ teaspoon salt
1 teaspoon vanilla extract
2 tablespoons butter or margarine

PIE FILLING

1 pint Peach "Ice Cream," softened (page 241)

1 cup fresh raspberries
2 medium ripe peaches, sliced
2 tablespoons honey or agave nectar
Fresh mint, for garnish

1. Grease 9-inch pie plate. Combine crust ingredients in bowl, then press mixture on bottom and up sides of prepared pie plate. Bake at 325°F for 10–15 minutes, until lightly toasted. Watch carefully so crust doesn't burn. Cool thoroughly.
2. Spread softened peach ice cream in cooled crust. Return to freezer for 4 hours, until firm. Remove from freezer 15 minutes before serving.
3. To prepare topping, wash and pick over fresh raspberries, combine with sliced peaches, and toss with honey. Top each serving with 1 tablespoon of peach-raspberry mixture. Garnish with sprig of fresh mint.

Nutrition Information (per serving)
Calories 210 • Fat 9g • Protein 2g • Carbohydrates 30g • Cholesterol 9mg • Sodium 161mg • Fiber 3g

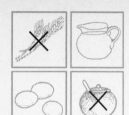

CHEESECAKE

Serves 12

This recipe is rich and creamy, but unfortunately it contains dairy and eggs. See the recipe on page 223 for dairy-free, egg-free cheesecake.

1 cup crushed Vanilla Wafers (page 235) or gluten-free cookies of choice

2 tablespoons softened butter or canola oil

1 cup dry-curd cottage cheese

3 large eggs

2 packages (8 ounces each) low-fat cream cheese, softened

1 teaspoon grated lemon zest

2 tablespoons fresh lemon juice

1 cup granulated sugar or fructose powder

1 tablespoon tapioca flour

¼ teaspoon salt

1½ teaspoons vanilla extract

Fresh strawberries or raspberries, for garnish (optional)

1. Coat bottom and sides of 8-inch springform pan with cooking spray. Combine vanilla wafers and butter in a blender and process until well mixed. Press crumbs onto bottom of prepared pan and slightly up sides. Refrigerate while preparing filling.

2. Preheat oven to 300°F. In food processor, puree cottage cheese and eggs for 3 minutes, or until silky smooth. Add remaining ingredients and puree until smooth. Pour into chilled crust.

3. Bake for 1 hour, until cheesecake is set. Cool in pan on wire rack. Cover and refrigerate up to 8 hours or overnight.

4. To serve, remove sides of pan and transfer cheesecake to serving plate. Garnish with fresh strawberries or raspberries, if desired.

Nutrition Information (per serving)
Calories 275 • Fat 13g • Protein 8g • Carbohydrates 32g • Cholesterol 74mg • Sodium 350mg • Fiber <1g

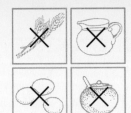

CHEESECAKE
WITHOUT EGGS

Serves 12

This recipe allows you to indulge in a slice of luscious, creamy cheesecake without dairy or eggs.

1 cup crushed Vanilla Wafers
(page 235) or gluten-free cookies
of choice

2 tablespoons softened butter or
canola oil

1 tablespoon honey or agave nectar

4 teaspoons unflavored gelatin powder

1 cup evaporated skim milk or soy milk

¾ cup granulated sugar or fructose
powder*

1 tablespoon vanilla extract

2 cups sour cream alternative or cream
cheese alternative**

1 cup Yogurt Cheese** (page 114)

Grated zest of 1 lemon

Fresh fruit of choice, for garnish (optional)

1. Preheat oven to 350°F. Grease 8-inch springform pan.
2. In food processor, process vanilla wafers until fine crumbs form. Add butter and honey and process again until well mixed. Remove crumbs and press onto bottom and up sides of prepared pan. Bake for 10–15 minutes. Set aside.
3. Stir gelatin into milk in small saucepan. Wait 1 minute, then heat gently on low heat about 3 minutes, until gelatin is dissolved.
4. In food processor, process sugar or fructose powder, vanilla, sour cream, and yogurt cheese or tofu until very smooth. Add lemon zest and gelatin mixture and pulse until well mixed. Pour into prepared crust and chill in refrigerator for 3 hours.
5. To serve, unmold by running a sharp knife around edge of pan. Slice with warm knife. Garnish with fresh fruit of choice, if desired.

Nutrition Information (per serving)
Calories 200 • Fat 8g • Protein 4g • Carbohydrates 30g • Cholesterol 15mg • Sodium 140mg • Fiber 0.5g

*Sugar Alternative: You can use ½ cup honey in place of ¾ cup granulated sugar. If so, reduce milk to ¾ cup.
**Dairy Alternative: You can use 2 cups soft silken tofu in place of sour cream or cream cheese alternative. Also, you can use 1 cup soft silken tofu in place of 1 cup Yogurt Cheese.

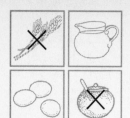

CHOCOLATE CHEESECAKE

Serves 10

This seems rich and creamy yet has fewer calories than expected. It is richer and creamier with whole milk or cream, but in this recipe I make it with 2% milk.

¼ cup crushed Chocolate Wafers
(page 229)

2 tablespoons softened butter or
canola oil

1 package (16 ounces) nonfat cream
cheese

1 cup cottage cheese (1% fat)

1 cup packed light brown sugar or
maple sugar

⅓ cup unsweetened cocoa powder
(not Dutch process)

½ cup tapioca flour

¼ cup 2% milk (cow, rice, or soy)

1 teaspoon vanilla extract

¼ teaspoon salt

1 large egg

2 tablespoons dairy-free, gluten-free
chocolate chips (optional)

Fresh fruit of choice, for garnish
(optional)

1. Preheat oven to 300°F. Grease 8-inch springform pan.
2. Combine chocolate wafers and butter in food processor and process until fine crumbs form. Sprinkle crumbs in bottom of prepared pan. Set aside.
3. In food processor, process cream cheese and cottage cheese until very, very smooth. Add brown sugar, cocoa powder, flour, milk, vanilla, and salt. Process mixture until smooth. Add egg and blend just until blended. Stir in chocolate chips (if using). Slowly pour mixture over crumbs in pan.
4. Bake for 1 hour, or until cheesecake is set. Cool in pan on wire rack. Cover and chill for at least 8 hours or overnight. Remove sides of pan and transfer cake to serving plate. Garnish with fresh fruit of choice, if desired.

Nutrition Information (per serving)
Calories 230 • Fat 11g • Protein 8g • Carbohydrates 25g • Cholesterol 40mg • Sodium 270mg • Fiber 2g

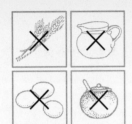

CHOCOLATE CHEESECAKE WITHOUT EGGS

Serves 12

This cheesecake has the same rich chocolate flavor as a traditional chocolate cheesecake but without eggs or dairy. Make sure the cream cheese alternative is appropriate for your diet.

1 cup crushed Chocolate Wafers
  (page 229)

2 tablespoons softened butter or
  canola oil

1 tablespoon honey or agave nectar

4 teaspoons unflavored gelatin powder

1 cup evaporated skim milk (or rice or
  soy milk)

½ cup unsweetened cocoa powder
  (not Dutch process)

¾ cup packed light brown sugar
  or maple sugar

2 teaspoons vanilla extract

1 teaspoon instant coffee powder
  (optional)

2 cups sour cream alternative or cream
  cheese alternative or soft silken tofu

1 cup Yogurt Cheese (page 114)
  or soft silken tofu

2 teaspoons grated orange zest
  (optional)

1. Preheat oven to 350°F. Grease 8-inch springform pan.
2. Place chocolate wafers in food processor and process until fine crumbs form. Add butter and honey and process again. Remove crumbs and press onto bottom and up sides of prepared pan. Bake for 10–15 minutes. Set aside.
3. Sprinkle gelatin over milk in small saucepan and soften 1 minute. Heat gently over low heat about 3 minutes, until gelatin dissolves. (If using maple sugar, dissolve in warmed milk after gelatin dissolves.)
4. In food processor, combine cocoa, sugar, vanilla, coffee powder (if using), sour cream or cream cheese, and yogurt cheese or tofu and process until very, very smooth. Add gelatin mixture and orange zest (if using) and process for 3 minutes, or until thoroughly mixed. Scrape sides of bowl down periodically. Pour into prepared crust and chill for 3 hours.
5. To serve, unmold and slice with warm knife. Garnish as desired.

Nutrition Information (per serving)

Calories 210 • Fat 9g • Protein 5g • Carbohydrates 30g • Cholesterol 15mg • Sodium 145mg • Fiber 2g

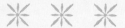

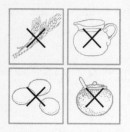

CHOCOLATE CHERRY ALMOND BISCOTTI

Makes 24 biscotti

Biscotti are an elegant treat meant for dipping into hot coffee, tea, or cappuccino. Though baked twice, they are extremely easy to make—especially if you mix the dough in a food processor.

1¾ cups Flour Blend (page 276)
1½ teaspoons xanthan gum
2 teaspoons baking powder
½ teaspoon salt
½ cup unsweetened cocoa powder
  (not Dutch process)
1 teaspoon instant coffee powder
¾ cup packed light brown sugar or
  maple sugar

2 large eggs, or ½ cup Flax Mix
  (page 108)
⅓ cup canola oil
1 teaspoon vanilla extract
½ teaspoon almond extract
¾ cup dried tart cherries
¼ cup gluten-free, dairy-free
  chocolate chips

1. Preheat oven to 350°F. Grease 17x11-inch baking sheet or line with parchment paper.
2. In food processor, combine flours, xanthan gum, baking powder, salt, cocoa, coffee powder, and sugar and process mixture until thoroughly blended. Add eggs, oil, vanilla, and almond extract. Process until dough forms a ball. Break ball into several pieces, add cherries, and process until dough forms ball again.
3. Divide dough in half. On baking sheet, shape each half into log measuring 2 inches wide by 12 inches long by ½ inch thick. Bake for 20 minutes. Remove from oven, but leave oven on.

4. Place each log on cutting board. (If using parchment paper, carefully slide parchment paper—logs and all—onto cutting board.) With electric knife or sharp, serrated knife, diagonally cut each log into ¾- to 1-inch slices. Place each slice on cut side. Return to oven, reduce heat to 275°F, and bake for 10 minutes. Turn slices over and bake for another 10 minutes.

5. To further crisp biscotti, turn oven off but leave baking sheet in oven for another 10–15 minutes with oven door closed.

6. For chocolate-dipped biscotti, melt chocolate in double boiler or heavy saucepan. Dip each piece halfway into melted chocolate. Place biscotti on waxed paper to cool. Store biscotti in an airtight container.

Nutrition Information (per cookie)

Calories 130 • Fat 5g • Protein 2g • Carbohydrates 24g • Cholesterol 1mg • Sodium 99mg • Fiber 1.5g

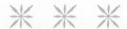

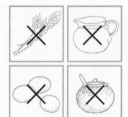

CHOCOLATE CHERRY COOKIES

Makes 16 cookies

Use dried cranberries instead of dried tart cherries for a different flavor twist.

¾ cup + 2 tablespoons Flour Blend (page 276)

1 teaspoon xanthan gum

½ cup unsweetened cocoa powder (not Dutch process)

1 teaspoon baking soda

¼ teaspoon salt

½ cup (1 stick) butter or margarine, at room temperature

½ cup granulated sugar

⅓ cup packed light brown sugar or maple sugar

1 large egg, or ¼ cup Flax Mix (page 108)

1 teaspoon vanilla extract

½ cup gluten-free, dairy-free chocolate chips

¼ cup dried tart cherries or cranberries

1. Preheat oven to 350°F. Grease baking sheet or line with parchment paper.
2. In medium mixer bowl, combine flours, xanthan gum, cocoa, baking soda, and salt.
3. With electric mixer, cream butter, sugars, egg, and vanilla until well combined. Add dry ingredients gradually and mix only until moistened. Fold in chocolate chips and cherries.
4. With small ice-cream scoop, place balls of dough (about 2 tablespoons each) 1 inch apart on prepared baking sheet.
5. Bake for 10–12 minutes, until puffed and cracked. Cool on baking sheet for 5 minutes, then transfer to wire rack to cool.

Nutrition Information (per cookie)
Calories 150 • Fat 7g • Protein 2g • Carbohydrates 22g • Cholesterol 24mg • Sodium 156mg • Fiber 1.5g

Chocolate Coconut Cookies: Add ¼ cup coconut flakes and ¼ cup chopped nuts (pecans, walnuts, or almonds). Bake as directed.

Calories 190 • Fat 10g • Protein 2g • Carbohydrates 26g • Cholesterol 27mg • Sodium 180mg • Fiber 2g

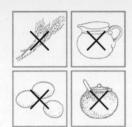

CHOCOLATE ICE-CREAM SANDWICHES

Serves 12 (2 wafers per serving)

These are so simple that your children or grandchildren can help make them. Be sure to buy ice cream that meets your dietary needs or make your own using the recipe on page 243.

CHOCOLATE WAFERS
¼ cup (½ stick) butter or margarine

2 tablespoons honey or agave nectar

½ cup packed light brown sugar or maple sugar

1 large egg, or ¼ cup Flax Mix (page 108)

1½ teaspoons vanilla extract

1⅓ cups Flour Blend (page 276)

¼ cup unsweetened cocoa powder (not Dutch process)

½ teaspoon xanthan gum

½ teaspoon salt

1½ teaspoons baking powder

FILLING & EDGES
1 pint ice cream of choice

1 cup chopped nuts of choice or crushed gluten-free, dairy-free chocolate chips or shredded coconut, for rolling edges of cookies

1. Preheat oven to 325°F. Grease nonstick baking sheet or line with parchment paper.
2. In food processor, combine butter, honey, sugar, egg, and vanilla until smooth. Add flours, cocoa, xanthan gum, salt, and baking powder and process until thoroughly combined. Shape batter into soft ball. Batter will be somewhat soft. Cover and refrigerate for 1 hour.
3. Shape dough into 24 balls (about 1 tablespoon each). Place balls on prepared baking sheet. Flatten each ball with a spatula to a 1½- to 2-inch circle, depending on preferred size of wafer. The wafers will spread more when butter is used and less when margarine is used.
4. Bake for 25–30 minutes, until wafers appear dry on top. Baking time depends on size of wafers; watch carefully so wafers don't burn.

5. To make sandwich wafers, place 2 tablespoons slightly softened ice cream between two wafers. Roll edges in chopped nuts, chocolate chips, or coconut. Freeze until ready to serve.

Nutrition Information (per serving for wafers only)
Calories 285 • Fat 14g • Protein 5g • Carbohydrates 40g • Cholesterol 35mg • Sodium 200mg • Fiber 2g

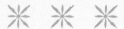

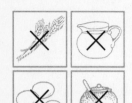

CHOCOLATE CHIP COOKIES

Makes 24 cookies

Chocolate chip cookies are every kid's favorite. Keep these on hand in the freezer and thaw a few when you need them.

1½ cups Flour Blend (page 276)
½ teaspoon baking soda
1 teaspoon xanthan gum
¼ teaspoon salt
¼ cup (½ stick) butter or margarine, at room temperature
¾ cup packed light brown sugar or maple sugar
⅓ cup granulated sugar or fructose powder

2 teaspoons vanilla extract
1 extra-large egg, or ¼ cup Flax Mix (page 108)
1 cup gluten-free, dairy-free chocolate chips
¼ cup chopped nuts of choice (optional)

1. Preheat oven to 350°F. Grease 13x9-inch nonstick baking sheet or line with parchment paper and set aside.
2. In mixer bowl, whisk together flours, baking soda, xanthan gum, and salt. Set aside.

3. In large mixer bowl, beat butter with brown sugar or granulated sugar or fructose powder, vanilla, and egg, scraping sides of bowl frequently. Beat in flour mixture on low speed, mixing thoroughly (or mix everything in a food processor).
4. Stir in chocolate chips and nuts (if using). Drop by tablespoonfuls on prepared baking sheet. (If you are using canola oil spread, the cookies won't spread as they bake. Press them down to ½-inch thickness with your palm or bottom of drinking glass. Use your fingers to shape cookie to a perfect circle.)
5. Bake on center rack of oven for 10–12 minutes, until lightly browned. Cool for 2–3 minutes before removing from baking sheet to wire rack to cool completely.

Nutrition Information (per cookie)
Calories 135 • Fat 5g • Protein 1g • Carbohydrates 24g • Cholesterol 13mg • Sodium 73mg • Fiber 0.5g

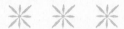

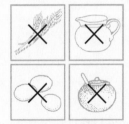

COLORADO CHOCOLATE CHIP COOKIES

Makes 24 cookies

There's nothing like a big fat chewy chocolate cookie—loaded with coconut, nuts, and fruit—to satisfy your chocolate cravings.

½ cup (1 stick) butter or margarine
½ cup packed light brown sugar or maple sugar
1 teaspoon vanilla extract
1 large egg, or ¼ cup Flax Mix (page 108)
¼ cup buttermilk, or ½ teaspoon vinegar or lemon juice and enough nondairy milk to equal ¼ cup

1¾ cups Flour Blend (page 276)
½ teaspoon baking soda
½ teaspoon salt
½ cup shredded coconut
½ cup chopped nuts of choice
½ cup dried tart cherries or cranberries
1½ cups gluten-free, dairy-free chocolate chips

1. Preheat oven to 350°F. Grease nonstick baking sheet or line with parchment paper.
2. In large mixer bowl, beat butter, sugar, and vanilla together until smooth. Beat in egg, then buttermilk.
3. In separate mixer bowl, combine flours, baking soda, and salt. Beat into egg mixture on low speed until incorporated.
4. Stir in coconut, nuts, cherries, and chocolate chips. Drop by tablespoonfuls (or use small spring-action ice-cream scoop for evenly sized cookies) onto prepared baking sheet.
5. Bake for 7–10 minutes, or until cookies are lightly puffed and slightly browned. Cool on wire rack. Store cookies in airtight container.

Nutrition Information (per cookie)
Calories 185 • Fat 10g • Protein 2g • Carbohydrates 26g • Cholesterol 18mg • Sodium 121mg • Fiber 1g

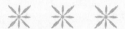

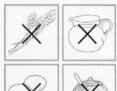

"OATMEAL" COOKIES

Makes 12 cookies

OK, so these aren't *really* oatmeal cookies, but they taste just as good. You'll find the rolled rice flakes in natural food stores. If not, order them from www.vitamin cottage.com or www.enjoylifefoods.com. Be sure to use potato flour—not potato starch or potato starch flour.

1⅓ cups Flour Blend (page 276)
½ cup packed light brown sugar
½ teaspoon salt
½ teaspoon xanthan gum
½ teaspoon baking soda
½ teaspoon baking powder
1 teaspoon ground cinnamon
1 large egg, or ¼ cup Flax Mix (page 108)

¼ cup (½ stick) butter or margarine
½ cup applesauce
2 tablespoons molasses or sorghum syrup
1 teaspoon vanilla extract
½ cup rolled rice flakes
¾ cup gluten-free, dairy-free chocolate chips or raisins

1. Preheat oven to 325°F. Grease nonstick baking sheet or line with parchment paper.
2. In mixer bowl, combine flours, sugar, salt, xanthan gum, baking soda, baking powder, and cinnamon.
3. In food processor, combine egg, butter, applesauce, molasses, and vanilla until well blended. Add flour mixture and rolled rice flakes and process until thoroughly mixed. Gently stir in chocolate chips or raisins. Dough will be somewhat stiff.
4. Drop by tablespoonfuls (or use small spring-action ice-cream scoop for evenly shaped cookies) onto prepared baking sheet. Flatten each cookie to ½-inch thickness with wet spatula.
5. Bake for 20–25 minutes, or until edges begin to brown. For a flavor twist, add ⅓ cup nut butter of your choice, such as almond, cashew, or soy.

Nutrition Information (per cookie)
Calories 210 • Fat 8g • Protein 2g • Carbohydrates 36g • Cholesterol 25mg • Sodium 239mg • Fiber 1.5g

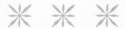

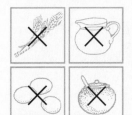

GINGERSNAPS

Makes 16 cookies

These freeze well, travel well, and make great crumb crusts for no-bake pies.

¼ cup (½ stick) butter or margarine

3 tablespoons molasses or sorghum syrup

½ cup packed light brown sugar or maple sugar

1 teaspoon vanilla extract

1½ cups Flour Blend (page 276)

1 teaspoon xanthan gum

½ teaspoon salt

1 teaspoon baking soda

1½ teaspoons ground ginger

1½ teaspoons ground cinnamon

¼ teaspoon ground nutmeg

¼ teaspoon ground cloves

2 tablespoons water (if needed)

Rice flour, for dusting

1. In food processor, combine butter, molasses, sugar, and vanilla. Add remaining ingredients and blend until dough forms a ball. (Add water, 1 tablespoon at a time, only if mixture fails to form a large ball—or if using electric mixer instead of food processor.) Refrigerate for 1 hour.
2. Preheat oven to 325°F. Grease baking sheet or line with parchment paper.
3. Dust your hands with rice flour and shape dough into 1-inch balls. Place on prepared baking sheet at least 1 inch apart. Flatten balls slightly with bottom of drinking glass.
4. Bake for 20–25 minutes, until cookies start to brown on bottom. Cool cookies on baking sheet for 5 minutes, then transfer to wire rack to cool completely. Store cookies in airtight container.

Nutrition Information (per cookie)
Calories 110 • Fat 3g • Protein 1g • Carbohydrates 26g • Cholesterol 0mg • Sodium 178mg • Fiber 0.5g

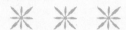

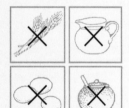

"GRAHAM" CRACKERS

Makes 24 crackers

These take a little work, but the kids in your family will especially appreciate your efforts.

½ cup brown rice flour or sorghum flour

½ cup soy flour

¼ cup tapioca flour

¼ cup potato starch

½ teaspoon xanthan gum

½ teaspoon salt

1 teaspoon baking powder

¾ teaspoon ground cinnamon

⅛ teaspoon *each* ground mace and ground ginger

⅓ cup packed light brown sugar or maple sugar

2 tablespoons honey or agave nectar

1 teaspoon vanilla extract

⅓ cup softened butter, margarine, or Spectrum spread

2 tablespoons water (or more if needed)

1. Place all ingredients in food processor and blend until mixture forms a ball. (Or mix ingredients with electric mixer, adding 1 tablespoon of water at a time until mixture can be shaped into a soft ball.) Refrigerate dough for 1 hour.
2. Preheat oven to 325°F. Grease nonstick baking sheet or line with parchment paper. Place dough on baking sheet and top with waxed paper or plastic wrap. Pat with your hands or roll to ⅛-inch thickness with rolling pin or tall glass. Remove paper and, using sharp knife, cut dough into 3-inch squares. Prick each square several times with a fork. (Or, roll dough onto parchment paper or nonstick silicone liners, cut squares, and transfer parchment paper or liner—with crackers on them—to baking sheet.)
3. Bake for 15–20 minutes, until brown, but watch carefully since the crackers burn easily. Remove crackers from oven when browned and run knife along cut lines again. Cool for 2 minutes on baking sheet, then cool on wire rack. Crackers become crisp as they cool.

Nutrition Information (per cracker)
Calories 70 • Fat 3g • Protein 1g • Carbohydrates 11g • Cholesterol 7mg • Sodium 87mg • Fiber 0.5g

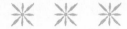

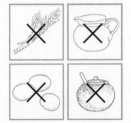

VANILLA WAFERS

Makes 16 wafers

This little cookie is very versatile and makes great snacks *and* great crumb crusts. Or just dunk them in your coffee.

¼ cup (½ stick) butter or margarine

2 tablespoons honey or agave nectar

3 teaspoons vanilla extract

1 cup Flour Blend (page 276)

½ cup sweet rice flour

½ cup packed light brown sugar or maple sugar

½ teaspoon xanthan gum

½ teaspoon baking soda

½ teaspoon salt

1 teaspoon vinegar

2 tablespoons water (if using an electric mixer)

Rice flour, for dusting

1. Blend all ingredients in food processor and process until mixture forms ball. Add water only if necessary (or if mixing with an electric mixer). Refrigerate for 1 hour.
2. Preheat oven to 325°F. Grease baking sheet or line with parchment paper.
3. With rice-floured hands, shape dough into 1-inch balls. Place on prepared baking sheet. Flatten each ball to ¼-inch thickness with bottom of drinking glass.
4. Bake for 20–25 minutes, until cookies are lightly browned. Remove from baking sheet and cool. Store cookies in airtight container. If cookies harden, place apple slice in covered container or gently warm in microwave oven.

Nutrition Information (per cookie)
Calories 130 • Fat 3g • Protein 1g • Carbohydrates 25g • Cholesterol 8mg • Sodium 157mg • Fiber 0.5g

Note: For a somewhat softer cookie, add egg yolk to ingredients in food processor.

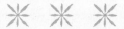

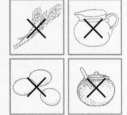

CHOCOLATE BROWNIES

Makes 12 brownies

This is one of my family's favorite recipes, and my guests love to be pampered with this all-American favorite.

1 cup Flour Blend (page 276)
⅔ cup unsweetened cocoa powder (not Dutch process)
½ teaspoon baking powder
½ teaspoon salt
1 teaspoon xanthan gum
⅓ cup butter or margarine, melted
½ cup packed light brown sugar or maple sugar

½ cup granulated sugar or fructose powder
1 large egg*
2 teaspoons vanilla extract
⅓ cup hot water or brewed coffee (110°F)
¼ cup chopped walnuts (optional)

1. Preheat oven to 350°F. Grease 8-inch square nonstick baking pan or 11x7-inch nonstick baking pan for a thinner brownie.
2. In mixer bowl, combine flours, cocoa, baking powder, salt, and xanthan gum. Set aside.
3. In large mixer bowl, beat butter, sugars, egg, and vanilla with electric mixer on medium speed until well blended. With mixer on low speed, add dry ingredients and hot water or coffee. Mix until just blended. Mixture will be somewhat thick. Stir in nuts (if using). Spread batter in prepared pan with wet spatula.
4. Bake for 20 minutes. Cool brownies before cutting.

Nutrition Information (per serving)
Calories 190 • Fat 7g • Protein 2g • Carbohydrates 34g • Cholesterol 29mg • Sodium 164mg • Fiber 2g

Double Chocolate Brownies: Add ⅓ cup gluten-free, dairy-free chocolate chips or finely chopped dark gluten-free, dairy-free chocolate to batter.

Calories 210 • Fat 8g • Protein 3g • Carbohydrates 37g • Cholesterol 29mg • Sodium 164mg • Fiber 2g

*Chocolate Brownies Without Eggs: Omit egg and add 2 teaspoons egg replacer powder when mixing dry ingredients. Increase hot water or coffee to ⅔ cup. Bake as directed.

Calories 180 • Fat 6g • Protein 2g • Carbohydrates 34g • Cholesterol 29mg • Sodium 107mg • Fiber 1.5g

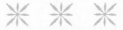

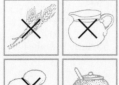
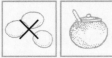

ROCKY ROAD BROWNIES

Serves 12

Absolutely and completely decadent—chocoholics will love this one. It's meant to be truly decadent. If nuts are not appropriate for your diet, omit them or substitute pumpkin seeds or sunflower seeds.

1¼ cups Flour Blend (page 276)

½ cup unsweetened cocoa powder (not Dutch process)

½ teaspoon baking powder

½ teaspoon salt

½ teaspoon xanthan gum

¼ cup (½ stick) butter or margarine or canola oil

½ cup granulated sugar or fructose powder

½ cup packed light brown sugar or maple sugar

1 large egg*

2 teaspoons vanilla extract

¼ cup warm water or coffee (110°F)

½ cup gluten-free, dairy-free chocolate chips or chopped chocolate squares

½ cup chopped pecans

½ cup miniature Kraft Jet-Puffed marshmallows

½ cup dried tart cherries or cranberries

1. Preheat oven to 350°F. Grease 8-inch square nonstick baking pan. In mixer bowl, stir together flours, cocoa, baking powder, salt, and xanthan gum and set aside.

2. In large mixer bowl, beat butter, sugars, and egg with electric mixer on medium speed until well combined.

3. With mixer on low speed, add dry ingredients. Mix until just blended; a few lumps may remain. Add vanilla and warm water or coffee and mix until thoroughly blended. Gently stir in chocolate chips, nuts, marshmallows, and cherries.

4. Spread batter in prepared pan and bake for 35 minutes. Cool brownies before cutting.

Nutrition Information (per serving)

Calories 255 • Fat 8g • Protein 3g • Carbohydrates 48g • Cholesterol 25mg • Sodium 153mg • Fiber 2g

***Rocky Road Brownies Without Eggs:** Omit egg and add 2 teaspoons egg replacer powder with dry ingredients. Increase water or coffee to ½ cup.

Calories 250 • Fat 8g • Protein 2g • Carbohydrates 48g • Cholesterol 10mg • Sodium 148mg • Fiber 2g

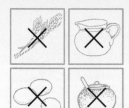

BASIC CUTOUT COOKIES

Makes 16 cookies

There are many uses for these versatile cookies.

¼ cup (½ stick) butter or margarine,
    at room temperature

2 tablespoons honey or agave nectar

½ cup granulated sugar or
    fructose powder

1 tablespoon vanilla extract

2 teaspoons grated lemon zest

1½ cups Flour Blend (page 276)

½ teaspoon xanthan gum

½ teaspoon salt

1 teaspoon baking powder

½ teaspoon baking soda

1 large egg white, or 2 tablespoons
    water or more (if needed)

Additional rice flour, for rolling

1. In food processor, combine butter, honey, sugar or fructose powder, vanilla, and lemon zest and process for 1 minute. Add flours, xanthan gum, salt, baking powder, and baking soda, and process until dough forms large clumps. Scrape down sides of bowl with spatula. Process until dough forms ball again. Add egg white or water if necessary, 1 tablespoon at a time. Refrigerate for 1 hour.

2. Preheat oven to 325°F. Grease baking sheet or line with parchment paper. Using half of dough, roll to ¼-inch thickness between sheets of waxed paper or plastic wrap sprinkled with rice flour. Keep remaining dough chilled until ready to use. Cut into desired shapes (about 2 inches in diameter) and transfer to prepared baking sheet.

3. Bake for 10–12 minutes, until cookies are lightly browned. Remove from baking sheet and cool on wire rack.

Nutrition Information (per cookie)
Calories 165 • Fat 6g • Protein 2g • Carbohydrates 28g • Cholesterol 8mg • Sodium 162mg •
    Fiber 0.5g

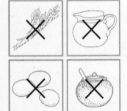

CHOCOLATE CAPPUCCINO "ICE CREAM"

Makes about 3 cups

The coffee flavor will be more pronounced if you use espresso rather than regular coffee.

½ cup packed light brown sugar or
    maple sugar
½ cup hot brewed espresso or very
    strong brewed coffee
2 packages (12 ounces each) soft
    silken tofu
2 tablespoons unsweetened cocoa
    powder (not Dutch process)

1 teaspoon vanilla extract
1 teaspoon espresso powder
    or instant coffee powder
½ teaspoon ground cinnamon
¼ teaspoon xanthan gum
⅛ teaspoon salt

1. Dissolve sugar in hot espresso. Add to food processor, along with remaining ingredients, and process until very smooth.
2. Cover and chill until mixture reaches 40°F. Freeze mixture in ice-cream maker, following manufacturer's directions.

Nutrition Information (per ½-cup serving)
Calories 130g • Fat 3g • Protein 5g • Carbohydrates 22g • Cholesterol 0mg • Sodium 63mg • Fiber 1g

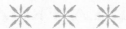

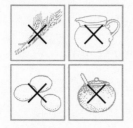

PEACH "ICE CREAM"

Makes 1 quart

Make this "ice cream" in the summer when peaches are in season. It's great alone or on a pie.

2 cups sliced fresh peaches
1 package (12 ounces) soft silken tofu
½ cup 2% milk (cow, rice, or soy)
½ cup granulated sugar or
    fructose powder
¼ cup fresh lemon juice

1 tablespoon butter or margarine
1 teaspoon vanilla extract
1 teaspoon almond extract
¼ teaspoon salt
¼ teaspoon xanthan gum

1. Place all ingredients in food processor and blend until very, very smooth. Chill mixture until it reaches 40°F.
2. Freeze mixture in ice-cream maker, following manufacturer's directions. When ready to serve, use a spring-action ice-cream scoop or melon baller to remove balls of ice cream. Serve immediately with your favorite sauce.

Nutrition Information (per ½-cup serving)
Calories 110 • Fat 3g • Protein 3g • Carbohydrates 20g • Cholesterol 4mg • Sodium 47mg •
  Fiber 1g

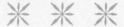

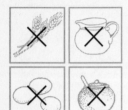

VANILLA FROZEN YOGURT

Makes 1 quart

One of America's favorite flavors, but without the eggs often found in frozen confections.

>   2 cups vanilla-flavored nonfat yogurt (cow or soy)
>   1¾ cups 2% milk (cow, rice, or soy)
>   ½ cup honey or agave nectar
>   3 teaspoons vanilla extract
>   2 teaspoons unflavored gelatin powder

1. Place all ingredients in food processor and process until very smooth. Chill mixture to 40°F.
2. Freeze mixture in ice-cream maker, following manufacturer's directions.

Nutrition Information (per ½-cup serving)
Calories 140 • Fat 1g • Protein 6g • Carbohydrates 29g • Cholesterol 4mg • Sodium 70mg • Fiber 0g

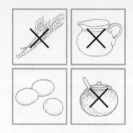

VANILLA "ICE CREAM" WITH EGGS

Makes 1 quart

This delicious frozen treat omits dairy, but it is the egg yolks that give it a creamy texture. So, it will be perfect for those *without* egg sensitivities.

   1 teaspoon unflavored gelatin powder
   4 cups milk (cow, rice, or soy), divided
   ½ cup honey or agave nectar
   4 large egg yolks, beaten until very smooth
   3 teaspoons vanilla extract

1. In mixer bowl, combine gelatin with 3 tablespoons milk and stir until dissolved. Add gelatin mixture, honey, and remaining milk to small saucepan. Cook over low heat until mixture almost boils. Remove from heat.

2. Whisk ½ cup of hot mixture into eggs. Add eggs to mixture in saucepan. Return saucepan to low-medium heat and cook, stirring, for 2 minutes. Do not boil; mixture may curdle. Remove from heat. Stir in vanilla. Refrigerate mixture until temperature reaches 40°F. Freeze mixture in ice-cream maker, following manufacturer's directions.

Nutrition Information (per ½-cup serving)
Calories 140 • Fat 3g • Protein 6g • Carbohydrates 24g • Cholesterol 109mg • Sodium 68mg •
   Fiber 0g

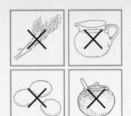

BUTTERSCOTCH PUDDING

Serves 4

This butterscotch pudding, one of my family's favorites, is a nice change from chocolate.

½ cup packed dark brown sugar or
    maple sugar

2 tablespoons cornstarch*

¼ teaspoon salt

1½ cups evaporated skim milk, or 1⅓
    cups 2%* milk (cow, rice,* or soy)

1 large egg yolk (optional)

1 tablespoon butter or
    margarine

1 teaspoon vanilla extract

½ teaspoon butter-flavored extract
    (optional)

1. Whisk together sugar, cornstarch, and salt in large, heavy saucepan over medium heat. Add milk gradually, whisking constantly. Whisk in egg yolk (if using) and bring mixture to boiling, whisking constantly.

2. Immediately reduce heat to low and continue to boil, stirring, for another full minute. (This boiling time is critical because it develops the caramel, butterscotch flavor—but be careful, mixture may splatter as it boils.)

3. Remove from heat and stir in butter, vanilla, and butter extract (if using). Divide among 4 small dessert cups and refrigerate for 2 hours.

Nutrition Information (per ½-cup serving)
Calories 160 • Fat 4g • Protein 8g • Carbohydrates 23g • Cholesterol 64mg • Sodium 270mg •
    Fiber 0g

*If using rice milk, increase cornstarch to 3 tablespoons.

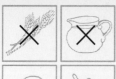

CHOCOLATE PUDDING

Serves 4

Of all the recipes in this book, I've probably made this one most often. It's my favorite comfort food and so quick to make. I often don't even wait for it to cool in the refrigerator. I just eat it while it's still warm because I can't wait any longer.

⅓ cup granulated sugar or maple sugar

2 tablespoons cornstarch*

2 tablespoons unsweetened cocoa powder (not Dutch process)

⅛ teaspoon salt

1¾ cups 2% milk (cow, rice,* or soy)

1 ounce gluten-free, dairy-free chocolate chips

1 teaspoon vanilla extract

In medium-size, heavy saucepan, whisk together sugar, cornstarch, cocoa powder, and salt. Gradually whisk in milk. Bring to boiling over medium heat, whisking constantly. Cook for 1 minute, stirring constantly. Remove pudding from heat and stir in chocolate chips until melted. Stir in vanilla. Chill.

Nutrition Information (per ½-cup serving)

Calories 180 • Fat 5g • Protein 4g • Carbohydrates 30g • Cholesterol 8mg • Sodium 132mg • Fiber 1g

*If using rice milk, increase cornstarch to 3 tablespoons.

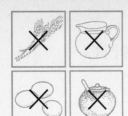

CHOCOLATE ESPRESSO POTS DE CRÈME

Serves 4

This is a very simple yet elegant dessert. Top with a dollop of whipped topping, a dusting of cinnamon, or fresh strawberries.

2 tablespoons unsweetened cocoa powder (not Dutch process)

½ cup packed light brown sugar or maple sugar

2 tablespoons + 1 teaspoon cornstarch*

1 teaspoon instant coffee or espresso powder

2 cups 2% milk (cow, rice,* or soy)

1 ounce gluten-free, dairy-free bittersweet or semisweet chocolate chips or pieces

¼ teaspoon salt

1 teaspoon vanilla extract

1. In medium saucepan, combine cocoa, sugar, cornstarch, and espresso. Over medium heat, add milk, chocolate, and salt, and cook about 5–8 minutes, whisking constantly until chocolate melts and mixture thickens.
2. Remove from heat; add vanilla. Pour into 4 individual dessert bowls. Chill until firm.

Nutrition Information (per serving)
Calories 200 • Fat 2g • Protein 5g • Carbohydrates 43g • Cholesterol 2mg • Sodium 222mg • Fiber 1g

*If using rice milk, increase cornstarch to 3 tablespoons.

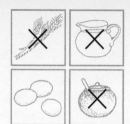

VANILLA CUSTARD

Serves 4

This recipe is versatile, but it contains eggs.

1 cup 2% milk (cow, rice, or soy)
½ cup granulated sugar or fructose powder
¼ cup cornstarch

4 large egg yolks, at room temperature
1 tablespoon butter, margarine, or canola oil
2 teaspoons vanilla extract

1. Heat milk to simmering (not boiling) in medium-size, heavy pan over medium-low heat. Set aside.
2. Meanwhile, mix sugar and cornstarch in small bowl. In another bowl, beat egg yolks with electric mixer until thick and lemon-colored. Slowly add cornstarch mixture to eggs, mixing until smooth. Gradually whisk into hot milk.
3. Return mixture to pan and cook for 2 minutes, whisking constantly, over low heat, until thickened. Remove from heat. Stir in butter and vanilla. Chill in bowl, covered with plastic wrap touching surface of custard.

Nutrition Information (per serving)
Calories 245 • Fat 10g • Protein 5g • Carbohydrates 30mg • Cholesterol 230mg • Sodium 67mg • Fiber 0g

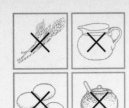

CHERRY PIE FILLING

Makes about 2 cups

Use this easy recipe when you don't want to use commercial cherry pie filling.

1 can (16 ounces) tart cherries
1 tablespoon tapioca flour
⅓ cup granulated sugar or
    fructose powder

¼ teaspoon salt
1 teaspoon vanilla extract
1 teaspoon almond extract
Dash red food coloring (optional)

1. Drain cherries, reserving ¼ cup juice. Combine reserved juice with tapioca flour until thoroughly blended.
2. Place tapioca mixture, cherries, sugar or fructose powder, and salt in glass or ceramic saucepan. Cook over medium heat until mixture thickens, stirring constantly. Remove from heat; stir in vanilla, almond extract, and red food coloring (if using). Cool before using.

Nutrition Information (per 2-tablespoon serving)
Calories 45 • Fat 0.5g • Protein 1g • Carbohydrates 11g • Cholesterol 0mg • Sodium 50mg •
    Fiber 1g

Appendix A

BAKING WITHOUT CONVENTIONAL INGREDIENTS

All conventional baked goods usually contain wheat flour, milk or dairy, eggs, cane sugar, and a leavening agent, and each ingredient plays a unique role in producing tasty, pleasingly textured results. What happens when we omit these ingredients? Let's take each separately.

WHEAT FLOUR

I'm often asked, "If you can't use wheat flour, what else is there?" Well, there are plenty of other flours. Instead of using wheat and gluten flours, the recipes in this book feature a variety of flours—sorghum, rice, corn, bean, potato starch, and tapioca. These flours are safest for the largest number of people, the flours are least likely to compete with the flavors of the dish, and combinations of these flours produce very pleasing results. In some recipes, however, I use other flours such as amaranth, Montina (Indian rice grass), and quinoa, since these flours are particularly nutritious in terms of protein and fiber and they lend some interesting variation to our diet.

In place of rice flour, many recipes use sorghum flour. Others use garbanzo/fava bean flour. This flour is ideal for people who want to increase their protein intake, provided they're not allergic to or intolerant of legumes. The flour does not alter the dish's flavor but does impart a slightly sweeter taste than rice flour. One caution: Avoid this flour if you have a condition called glucose-6-phosphate dehydrogenase (G6PD) deficiency in which fava beans cause digestive problems.

Baking without wheat flour produces a somewhat heavier and denser product because the missing gluten can't establish a cell structure in which the leavening agent does its job. However, using xanthan gum helps alleviate this situation to the extent that many people can't distinguish between cakes made with or without wheat flour. Each recipe that requires xanthan gum tells you exactly how much to use for optimum results.

I'm often asked about exchanging potato starch for cornstarch and vice versa. In place of potato starch, cornstarch can be substituted in a 1:1 ratio—assuming you can eat corn. Or, use 1 cup of amaranth starch. And 1 cup of tapioca flour can be replaced with ⅞ cup sweet rice flour.

BAKING WITH WHEAT-FREE FLOURS

The following tables and related discussion are designed to help you better understand the different gluten-free flours in terms of baking characteristics, color and flavor, general comments, and storage recommendations.

FLOUR	TRAITS
Almond	
Baking	Made from ground almonds; sometimes called almond meal. If you grind your own flour from almonds, be sure to grind it as fine as possible. Produces baked goods with lovely golden color. Use almond flour as 25–33% of total flour blend.
Color and Flavor	Light-colored flour; has nutty, almond flavor.
General Comments	Provides good fiber content.
Storage	Has a high-fat content, so refrigerate to avoid rancidity.
Amaranth	
Baking	Especially good in dark-colored baked goods or those with spices such as chocolate cakes or cookies, spice cakes, and dark breads. Tends to brown quickly. Best when blended with other flours as no more than 15–20% of blend.
Color and Flavor	Mild, grainlike, nutty. Color varies from beige to nearly black, but usually light tan.

FLOUR	TRAITS
General Comments	Not related to wheat or other grains, it was cultivated by the Aztecs long ago. Color varies depending on origin. Higher in protein and fiber than any other grain. (Amaranth starch is starch of the amaranth seed and can be used as a 1:1 ratio replacement for cornstarch or potato starch.)
Storage	Airtight container in cool, dry, dark place. Refrigeration preferred, since flavor may intensify or turn rancid during prolonged storage. Buy in small quantities to avoid aging.

Arrowroot

Baking	Good in baking because it adds no flavor of its own and lightens baked goods. If used as breading, produces golden brown crust.
Color and Flavor	Snow-white in color—looks like cornstarch. Flavorless.
General Comments	Silky, fine powder. Often used to replace cornstarch or tapioca flour.
Storage	Airtight container in cool, dry, dark place.

Bean

Baking	Three kinds of bean flour: (1) white bean flour, (2) pure garbanzo or chickpea flour, and (3) blend of garbanzo flour and fava bean flour available from Authentic Foods, Bob's Red Mill, and Ener-G Foods. (See Mail-Order Sources in Resources section at back of book). Bean flours provide protein that is beneficial in baking. Use in combination with other flours to totally (or partially) replace rice flour.
Color and Flavor	Light tan or yellowish. Slight "beany" flavor, especially if flour is pure chickpeas or garbanzo bean—less so if using garbanzo/fava bean combination. The latter gives slightly sweet taste to baked goods.
General Comments	Adds important protein to otherwise "starchy" gluten-free flour blends.
Storage	Airtight container in cool, dry, dark place.

FLOUR	TRAITS
Chestnut	
Baking	Lends a silky texture and nutty flavor. Don't confuse it with water chestnut flour, which is quite starchy. Should be used with other flours (up to 25% of the blend in baking).
Color and Flavor	Ground from chestnuts, this is a light beige flour.
General Comments	Also called marrons, chestnuts are lower in fat than other nuts.
Storage	Store in dark, dry place.
Corn	
Baking	Excellent in corn bread, muffins, and waffles—especially when blended with cornmeal. Corn flour is finely ground cornmeal, which you can grind yourself. Or use Shiloh Farms brand corn flour. (See Mail-Order Sources in Resources section at back of book.)
Color and Flavor	Light yellow or white in color. Tastes like corn.
General Comments	Smooth flour from corn.
Storage	Airtight container in cool, dry, dark place.
Cornmeal	
Baking	Excellent in corn bread, muffins, and waffles—especially when blended with corn flour. Blue cornmeal can be substituted in muffins and waffles.
Color and Flavor	White or yellow. Tastes like corn. Blue cornmeal is grayish blue and has a somewhat stronger flavor.
General Comments	Coarser than corn flour; often used in Mexican dishes. Used in polenta but is often a coarser grind than regular cornmeal. Blue cornmeal can substitute for white or yellow cornmeal in some Mexican dishes.
Storage	Airtight container in cool, dry, dark place.

FLOUR	TRAITS
Indian Rice Grass	
Baking	Commercially marketed as Montina. Relatively high in protein, it works best blended with other, lighter flours. Use as 25% of the flour blend.
Color and Flavor	Light brown/gray color. Produces darker-colored baked goods with a hearty "wheatlike" flavor and pleasant "chew" due to higher fiber content.
General Comments	This flour, developed from Indian rice grass, is grown in Montana. Available at www.amazinggrains.com
Storage	Store in cool, dry, dark place. Or refrigerate, tightly covered.
Mesquite	
Baking	Comes in flour and meal versions. Wonderful in baked desserts such as cakes, cookies, and brownies. Best when used as 25% of the flour blend.
Color and Flavor	Light tan color; slightly sweet, nutty flavor with a hint of molasses. Lends a brown tint to baked goods, so it's best in darker-colored foods.
General Comments	Derived from the pods of mesquite trees, whose branches are used in mesquite grilling. Believed to stabilize blood sugar.
Storage	Airtight container in cool, dry, dark place.
Millet	
Baking	Lends a light yellow tint to baked goods and produces a light, dry crumb with a smooth, thin crust. Millet performs best when blended with other flours, comprising no more than 25% of the flour blend.
Color and Flavor	Light yellow color with mild, slightly cornlike flavor.
General Comments	Very high in protein but—due to its high alkalinity—one of the easier grains to digest.
Storage	Refrigerate, tightly covered, for 2 months. Purchase millet flour in small amounts and use it quickly because it can become bitter and rancid.

FLOUR	TRAITS
Potato Flour	
Baking	Use in very small quantities in baking; adds crispness and density, or "tooth," to baked goods.
Color and Flavor	Heavy, light-tan flour made from whole potatoes, including the skins. Slight potato flavor.
General Comments	Often mistaken for potato starch, but performs quite differently in baking.
Storage	Airtight container in refrigerator to prevent rancidity.
Potato Starch	
Baking	Excellent baking properties, especially when combined with eggs. Lumps easily, so stir with whisk before measuring.
Color and Flavor	Very white, fine powder. Bland flavor.
General Comments	Very fine, powdery texture. Made from the dried starch of potatoes. Not the same as potato flour, which is made from dried and ground whole potatoes. Potato flour is heavy and used very little in wheat-free cooking.
Storage	Airtight container in cool, dry, dark place.
Quinoa (keen-wah)	
Baking	Excellent in all types of baking, including cakes, cookies, breads, and biscuits. Best if blended with other flours (no more than 25%) and used in highly spiced or flavored foods.
Color and Flavor	Grain looks like sesame seeds. Flour color ranges from hues of red-yellow-orange to pink-purple-black, although flour tends to be tan. Flavor is somewhat nutty and can dominate baked goods.
General Comments	Not actually a cereal grain, but a member of the Chenopodiaceae family (related to beets and spinach). It is a complete protein and originally grown by the Incas of Peru.
Storage	Airtight container in cool, dry, dark place. Keeps well.

FLOUR	TRAITS
Rice (White or Brown)	
Baking	A bit gritty by itself, but works fine when combined with other flours. Should be about ⅔ of total flour. The coarser the grind, the more liquid needed.
Color and Flavor	White rice flour is white; brown rice flour has slight tan tint. Bland, pleasant-tasting flavor.
General Comments	Milled from broken hulls of rice kernel. Among least "allergenic" of all flours. Mostly starch and nutritionally inferior since bran and germ layers have been removed in milling.
Storage	Airtight container in cool, dry, dark place. Refrigerate brown rice flour to avoid rancidity.
Sorghum	
Baking	Works very well in all kinds of baking, especially bread. Best if blended with other flours, but can comprise up to 50% of flour blend.
General Comments	Newer, table sorghum variety is grown for human consumption (also called white food sorghum).
Storage	Store in airtight container in dark, dry, cool place.
Soy	
Baking	Excellent. Works well in baked goods with nuts, fruits, or chocolate. Best when combined with other flours, such as rice.
Color and Flavor	Yellow in color. Bland, somewhat nutty flavor—leans toward "beany." Flavor can be camouflaged by mixing with spices, fruit, nuts, or chocolate.
General Comments	Makes crispy coating for breading. Higher in protein and fat than other flours. Short shelf life, so purchase in small amounts to avoid spoilage. A common allergen, so use soy cautiously.
Storage	Airtight container in cool, dry, dark place. Best if refrigerated.

FLOUR	TRAITS

Sweet Potato

Baking	Produces baked goods with a great taste and texture. Its faint sweetness, however, will affect gravies and other savory sauces.
Color and Flavor	Light orange-yellow-colored flour with a faintly sweet taste.
General Comments	Ground from sweet potatoes, this hard-to-find flour is available in some specialty stores and at Ener-G Foods, www.Ener-G.com. (See Mail-Order Sources in Resources section at back of book.) A member of the morning glory family, sweet potatoes are one of the least allergenic foods on earth and a good choice for people with multiple sensitivities.
Storage	Refrigerate, tightly covered.

Sweet Rice

Baking	Don't confuse with white rice flour. Manufacturers suggest using in muffins, breads, and cakes although some sources recommend using only small amounts. Adds a nice elasticity to baked goods such as pie crusts.
Color and Flavor	White; bland in flavor. Easily confused with white rice flour because they look alike.
General Comments	Sometimes called sticky rice; often used in Chinese cooking. Contains more starch than rice flours, making it an excellent thickener. Helps inhibit separation of sauces when they're chilled or frozen.
Storage	Airtight container in cool, dark, dry place.

Tapioca

Baking	Excellent in baked products when it makes up 25–50% of total flour blend. Lightens baked goods and imparts "chewiness" to breads. Browns quickly and produces crispy coating in breading.
Color and Flavor	Snow-white, velvety powder. Anonymous flavor.

FLOUR	TRAITS
General Comments	Sometimes called cassava or cassava starch. Similar to arrowroot and can be used interchangeably.
Storage	Airtight container in cool, dark, dry place.
Teff	
Baking	A little gritty, but works well in baked goods such as cakes or breads—if used as 25–50% of total flour blend. Best in dark baked goods such as chocolate cake or brownies, pumpernickel bread, or gingerbread.
Color and Flavor	Brown color. Slightly strong tasting.
General Comments	Belongs to a tribe of its own in the grain family.
Storage	Airtight container in cool, dark, dry place.

Note: Ask your health professional if these alternatives are safe for your diet.

In place of 1 tablespoon wheat flour as thickener, use the following:

INGREDIENT	TRAITS	SUGGESTED USES
Agar (Kanten)		
1½ teaspoons	Use package directions. Colorless and flavorless. Sets at room temperature. Gels acidic liquids. Thin sauces need less.	Puddings, pie fillings, gelatin desserts, ice cream, glazes, cheese. Holds moisture and improves texture in pastry products.
Arrowroot		
1½ teaspoons	Mix in cold water first. Thickens at lower temperature. Don't boil. Add during last 5 minutes of cooking. Serve immediately. Clear, shiny. Semisoft when cool.	Any food requiring clear, shiny sauce, but good for egg or starch dishes where high heat is undesirable. Gives appearance of oil even if none used.

INGREDIENT	TRAITS	SUGGESTED USES
Bean Flour		
3 teaspoons	Produces yellowish, rich-looking sauce.	Soups, stews, gravies, but lends bean flavor.
Cornstarch		
1½ teaspoons	Mix in cold water first. Stir just until boiling. Makes clear, shiny sauce. Firms when cool.	Puddings, pie fillings, fruit sauces, soups. Gives appearance of oil even if none used.
Gelatin Powder		
1½ teaspoons	Dissolve in cold water, then heat until liquid is clear before using.	Gelatin puddings, aspics, cheesecakes. Won't gel acids like fresh pineapple.
Guar Gum		
1½ teaspoons	Mix with liquid first.	Large amounts are laxative.
Kudzu (Kuzu) Powder		
¾ teaspoon	Dissolve in cold water first. Odorless, tasteless. Makes smooth, transparent, soft sauces.	Puddings, pie fillings, and other dishes that must have "gelatin-like" consistency.
Quick-cooking Tapioca		
2 teaspoons	Mix with fruit, let stand 15 minutes before baking.	Fruit pies, cobblers, and tapioca pudding.
Rice Flour (Brown or White)		
1 tablespoon	Mix with cold liquid first. Somewhat grainy and coarse.	Soups, stews, or gravies or hearty, robust sauces.

INGREDIENT	TRAITS	SUGGESTED USES
Sweet Rice Flour		
1 tablespoon	Excellent thickener. Called glutinous rice.	Vegetable sauces and soups. (Has no wheat gluten.)
Tapioca Flour		
1½ tablespoons	Mix with cold water first. Add during last 5 minutes of cooking. Produces transparent, shiny sauce. Thick, soft gel when cool.	Soups, stews, gravies, potato dishes.
Xanthan Gum		
1 teaspoon	Mix with dry ingredients first; add to recipe.	Puddings, salad dressings, and gravies.

Note: Ask your health professional if these alternatives are safe for your diet.

WHEAT FLOUR EQUIVALENTS

Use the following table to convert your own recipes to gluten-free—or to modify recipes in this book. Be sure to use a blend of flours rather than just a single flour. Each of the flours has unique characteristics that affect the texture, taste, and appearance of baked goods.

Flours from reputable sources usually measure consistently time after time, although differences in flour-milling processes may affect consistency and texture. As you become more experienced with these flours, you can judge if the dough is too dry, too moist, or just right.

In place of 1 cup wheat flour, use:

FLOUR	AMOUNT
Amaranth Flour	1 cup
Buckwheat Flour	⅞ cup
Corn Flour	1 cup
Cornmeal	¾ cup
Cornstarch	¾ cup
Garbanzo (Chickpea) Flour	¾ cup
Garbanzo/Fava Bean Flour	1 cup
Indian Rice Grass (Montina)	1 cup
Mesquite Flour	1 cup
Millet Flour	1 cup
Nuts (Finely Ground)	½ cup
Potato Starch	¾ cup
Quinoa Flour	1 cup
Rice Flour (Brown/White)	⅞ cup
Sorghum Flour	1 cup
Soy Flour	½ cup + ½ cup potato starch
Sweet Rice Flour	⅞ cup
Tapioca Flour	1 cup
Teff Flour	⅞ cup

Note: Ask your health professional if these alternatives are safe for your diet.

Dairy

People avoid dairy products for three reasons: (1) allergies, (2) lactose intolerance, or (3) veganism. If lactose intolerance is your concern, you may use lactose-reduced milk in place of regular milk in these recipes. If you are allergic to dairy products or just want to avoid all dairy products for personal reasons, there are suggestions in each recipe for using milk substitutes made from rice, soy, potato, or nut milk.

Using milk substitutes is quite easy and usually has a minimal impact on the final product. In fact, most nondairy milks can be used interchangeably with cow's milk in baking. Each type of milk has a subtle taste and may produce slight color variations in the finished product (for example, soy milk may darken the product during baking).

Be sure to read the label on milk substitutes to make sure no other offending ingredients are present, such as barley malt extract, which is used to sweeten the milk. Sometimes a company will use one set of ingredients in the plain version yet another set of ingredients in the vanilla or chocolate version. Read the label each time you purchase the milk in case the manufacturing process or the ingredients change.

According to the Food Allergy & Anaphylaxis Network (FAAN) (www.foodallergy. org), people with milk allergies should avoid goat milk, goat yogurt, and goat cheeses, since the proteins are believed to be similar to those in products made from cow's milk. Some people with lactose intolerance say they can tolerate goat products, but the FAAN does not recommend this. Ask your physician to find out what's right for you.

People on a gluten-free diet must avoid oat milk—not because oats inherently contain gluten, but because of the possibility of contamination with wheat during the growing or manufacturing process.

There are also dairy-free yogurts and sour cream, but make sure they don't contain additional problem ingredients. For example, some items labeled "dairy-free" actually contain casein, a milk protein that must be avoided by milk-allergic people. Baking with other types of dairy substitutes such as cheese, sour cream, or cream cheese is more challenging, but the directions in the recipe will tell you how to handle the situation.

Baking with Dairy Substitutes

Milk is one of the easiest ingredients to make substitutions for in baking, although some milk substitutes lend a subtle flavor to baked goods and may affect the degree of browning while baking. In addition, read labels to avoid problem ingredients such as casein, which can be present even in food labeled "dairy-free," or barley malt, which contains gluten. Choose low-sugar versions when making savory dishes.

The suggestions offered in the following tables and related discussion on dairy substitutes are primarily for baking. However, the same amount of milk beverage substitute such as rice, soy, potato, or nut milk can be used in nonbaked items—like milk shakes, puddings, ice cream, or smoothies.

In place of 1 cup cow's milk, use:

SUBSTITUTE	AMOUNT TO USE	WHEN TO USE
Coconut Milk		
	Very high in fat unless you use the low-fat version. Not tested with baked goods in this book. However, many people use coconut milk successfully.	
Goat Milk		
Available in powder and liquid forms (and low-fat liquid) by Meyenberg. Not for milk allergies or lactose-intolerant.	1 cup. Most closely resembles cow's milk in color (pure white).	Any recipe. Works especially well in ice cream, puddings, and other milk-based dishes. Aseptic and powdered varieties have stronger flavor.
Nut Milk (Hazelnut or Almond)		
Not for nut allergies or intolerances.	1 cup. Mild, slightly nutty flavor. Light brown color.	Best in dessert recipes. May taste slightly "off" in savory dishes.
Oat Milk		
	May contain gluten. Not recommended for those with gluten intolerance.	

SUBSTITUTE	AMOUNT TO USE	WHEN TO USE
Rice Milk (Rice Beverage)		
Choose fortified, gluten-free brands.	1 cup. Mild flavor, white color. Looks like skim milk from cows.	Any recipe, but slightly sweet tasting. Reduce by 2 tablespoons per cup if used as buttermilk substitute.
Soy Milk (Soy Beverage)		
Choose fortified, gluten-free brands.	1 cup. Slight soy flavor, light tan in color. Buy in liquid or powder form and mix with water. Powdered version makes lighter-colored milk.	Best in recipes with stronger flavors to mask soy and in baked goods with darker colors since soy milk may darken with heat.

In place of 1 cup evaporated skim milk, use:

SUBSTITUTE	AMOUNT TO USE	WHEN TO USE
Ener-G Nut-Quik or Soy-Quik or other nondairy milk powder.	1 cup. Mix at double strength by using twice as much powder.	Recipes using evaporated skim milk. Flavors are stronger. Calories and nutrients will double.

In place of 1 cup buttermilk, use:

SUBSTITUTE	AMOUNT TO USE	WHEN TO USE
Use 1 tablespoon fresh lemon juice or cider vinegar and enough rice, soy, or nut milk to equal 1 cup.	1 cup. Some nondairy milks such as rice milk produce thinner buttermilk. If so, use 2 tablespoons less nondairy buttermilk per cup specified in recipe.	Any recipe calling for buttermilk.

If Recipe Calls for Dry Milk Powder: Use the same amount of nondairy milk powder by Solait, Better Than Milk, English Bay, or Vance's DariFree. Some brands are available in both soy and rice forms. Read labels to avoid problem ingredients such as casein. Or omit dry milk powder and add same amount of almond flour (finely ground blanched almonds). Baked goods won't brown as much without dry milk powder. In yeast breads, rising and browning are diminished without dry milk powder.

Density of Milk: Reduce liquid by 1 tablespoon per cup if using skim milk instead of whole milk, or very thin rice milk instead of a thicker version. Liquid milk varies by brand. The ratio of powder to water will affect the density of milk made from nondairy powders. Also, increase the thickener by 25 percent when rice milk is used in recipes that are thickened, such as pudding. Note that plain milk in a particular brand may contain one set of ingredients but flavored versions may contain different ingredients.

Lactose-Reduced Milk: Lactose-reduced milk may be used in these recipes. Be certain to read labels to avoid other offending ingredients. Also, some recipes may not produce the same results as those with "regular" cow's milk or nondairy milks.

Note: Ask your health professional if these alternatives are safe for your diet.

In place of 1 cup yogurt, use:

SUBSTITUTE	AMOUNT TO USE	WHEN TO USE
Goat Yogurt		
Not for people with milk allergies or lactose intolerance.	1 cup	Any recipe calling for yogurt. However, tapioca or other fillers in some goat yogurt may make the baked item "doughy."
Milk or Other Liquid		
(nut, soy, rice, or potato)	⅔ cup	Any recipe calling for yogurt. Best to add liquid in ⅓-cup increments to avoid adding too much.
Soy Yogurt		
	1 cup	Doesn't bake well, but use in dips, ice cream, and other nonbaked items. Won't drain.

Cheese: Although there are several "nondairy" cheeses such as Parmesan cheese made from rice or soy, it is difficult to find one that doesn't have additional problem ingredients. For example, they may contain milk proteins called calcum caseinate, sodium caseinate, or casein. Others include oats (which is off-limits for celiacs). Read the labels carefully to make sure the ingredients are appropriate for your situation.

Sour Cream and Cream Cheese: Soyco makes a rice-based version, but check the label for problem ingredients—the milk protein, casein, is present in both items. Soymage makes a casein-free sour cream alternative. Tofutti makes casein-free sour cream and cream cheese.

Note: Ask your health professional if these alternatives are safe for your diet.

EGGS

Eliminating eggs has as dramatic an impact on baking as omitting wheat flour. In fact, eliminating wheat flour and eggs are the two biggest challenges to allergy-free baking. Eggs not only bind ingredients and provide moisture, they are also leavening agents. This is the function we miss the most in baking. Several other ingredients can bind and moisturize a recipe, but eliminating eggs produces baked goods that are decidedly heavier and denser. For example, a cake that is light and airy when made *with* eggs becomes more like pound cake when made without eggs—but it is still delicious!

My favorite substitutes for eggs in baking are soft silken tofu and flaxseed meal, but there are other options as well. If you must avoid eggs, each recipe will tell you the best substitute to use.

BAKING WITH EGG SUBSTITUTES

Eggs are one of the hardest ingredients to exclude because they play such critical roles in baking. They are binding agents (hold ingredients together), moisturizers (add moisture), or leavening agents (make things rise). Generally speaking, egg-free baked goods don't rise as much and have a denser texture. Here are some general guidelines when cooking without eggs.

Eggs as Binders: If a recipe has only one egg but contains a fair amount of baking powder or baking soda, then the egg is the binder.

In place of 1 large egg as a binder, use:

SUBSTITUTE	AMOUNT TO USE	WHEN TO USE
Arrowroot, Soy, Lecithin		
(liquid or granular lecithin)	Mix ¼ cup warm water, 2 tablespoons arrowroot, 1 tablespoon soy flour, and ¼ teaspoon lecithin.	Stronger-flavored dishes since soy flour and lecithin may affect overall taste of dish.

SUBSTITUTE	AMOUNT TO USE	WHEN TO USE
Flaxseed Mix		
(brown or golden seeds or ground flax meal). Refrigerate all flax products.	¼ cup flax mix. Soak 1 teaspoon ground flaxseed in ¼ cup boiling water 5 minutes. Bake 25°F dishes slightly longer; lower temperature. Reduce oil by 1–2 tablespoons for every ¼ cup flaxseed mix used.	Cool before using. Best in dark-colored dishes. Mild flavor. Baked goods heavier, denser. Best in cookies, bars. Slight laxative.
Pureed Fruits or Vegetables		
Baby food without fillers (apples, pears)	3 tablespoons to replace each egg. Increase liquid in recipe by 1 tablespoon.	Baked goods where puree flavor complements or doesn't detract from dish's flavor.
Tofu		
(soft silken by Mori-Nu)	¼ cup for each egg. Blend with recipe liquid until very smooth.	Cakes, cookies, breads. Baked goods won't brown as deeply, but they will be very moist and some-what heavy.
Unflavored Gelatin Powder		
Knox or Grayslake brand	Mix 1 envelope gelatin in 1 cup boiling water. Use 3 tablespoons for each egg. Refrigerate the leftover mixture.	Baked goods such as cookies, cakes, breads. Microwave leftover mixture to liquefy.

Note: Ask your health professional if these alternatives are safe for your diet.

Liquid Egg Substitutes: You may use liquid egg substitutes in place of fresh eggs, but they still contain eggs. The yolks have been removed to reduce fat and cholesterol. *People with egg allergies must not eat these products because they still contain eggs. Also, some egg substitutes contain other problem ingredients for your diet. Always* read the label.

Eggs as Leavening Agents: If there are no other ingredients to make baked item rise, then the egg is the leavening agent.

In place of 1 egg as leavener, use:

SUBSTITUTE	AMOUNT TO USE	WHEN TO USE
Buttermilk, Yogurt, or Baking Soda		
	Replace recipe liquid with same amount of buttermilk or thinned yogurt. Replace baking powder with ¼ as much baking soda.	All baked goods; works best in dishes that don't need to rise a lot, such as cookies, bars, and flatbreads.
Egg Replacer Powder		
by Ener-G or Kingsmill	Ener-G suggests 1½ teaspoons powder mixed in 2 tablespoons water. I recommend 2–3 times as much powder in the same amount of water for better results.	All baked goods. Flavorless; won't affect taste of recipe. For added lightness, whip in food processor or blender for 30 seconds.

Other Hints When Omitting Eggs (if eggs are the leavening agent):

1. Add air to lighten the recipe by creaming the fat and sweetener together with an electric mixer. Then add dry ingredients.
2. Whip the liquid ingredients in a food processor or blender for 30 seconds.
3. Add an extra ½ teaspoon baking powder per egg, not to exceed 1 teaspoon baking powder per cup of flour. Too much baking powder may produce a bitter taste.
4. Recipes with acidic liquid such as buttermilk, molasses, lemon juice, or vinegar tend to rise better than those with nonacidic liquid such as water or milk.

Note: Ask your health professional if these alternatives are safe for your diet.

Eggs as Moisturizer: The egg's purpose is to add moisture if there are leavening agents in the recipe, but not much water or other liquid.

Generally speaking, baked goods without eggs are somewhat heavier and more dense. Slightly increase the leavening agent in egg-free recipes to compensate for the egg's natural leavening effect. In addition, using liquid sweeteners such as honey or molasses for part of the sugar in a recipe helps compensate for the loss of the "binding" effect of eggs.

In place of 1 egg as moisturizer, use:

SUBSTITUTE	AMOUNT TO USE	WHEN TO USE
Fruit Juice, Milk, or Water		
	2 tablespoons. Increase leavening by 25–50%. Bake items slightly longer, if necessary.	Baked goods such as cakes, cookies, bars.
Pureed Fruit		
Bananas, applesauce, apricots, pears, prunes. (The natural pectin in fruits, especially prunes, traps air, which helps "lighten" baked goods.)	¼ cup. Increase leavening by 25–50%. Bake items slightly longer, if necessary.	Baked goods where the fruit's flavor complements the overall dish such as applesauce in spice cakes, bananas in banana bread, apricots and pears in mild-flavored dishes, and prunes in dark, heavily flavored dishes such as chocolate cake or spice cake.

Note: Ask your health professional if these alternatives are safe for your diet.

CANE SUGAR

Baking with alternative sweeteners is both creative and challenging. It is creative because it's fun to see what different sweeteners bring to the baked dish in terms of taste and texture. For example, have you ever noticed that the cookies you buy in the bakeries at health food stores are usually soft and moist? That's because they're often sweetened with honey or fruit juices, rather than cane sugar. Honey and fruit juices are humectants; that is, they attract moisture, making the cookie soft and moist.

Baking with alternative sweeteners is also quite challenging. We don't realize it, but just like we associate wheat flavor with breads, our taste buds come to expect a certain flavor from sweeteners. And, although we think of sugar as fairly neutral in taste, it actually imparts a distinct flavor to baked goods that is hard to identify—until we bake without it. Then we know it's missing because there is a new flavor—and possibly a different texture—in its place, delivered by the new sweetener. But one of the joys of using substitutes is discovering new flavors that may eventually become our favorite flavors.

As I pointed out earlier, removing or even reducing the sugar in any baked item can affect its taste, texture, and appearance. Sugar is not only a flavor enhancer, but it also softens and tenderizes the crumb in baking. In addition, the sucrose in sugar produces the somewhat shiny, slightly crispy exterior we see on cakes and cookies, and it encourages nice, even browning, which gives baked goods their "finished" appearance.

Baked goods made without cane sugar will lack this shiny surface and won't brown as nicely. So, if you choose to bake with an alternative sweetener, be prepared for a slightly different-looking—and tasting—product.

BAKING WITH ALTERNATIVE SWEETENERS

This section on alternative sweeteners is divided into liquid sweeteners and granulated sweeteners. I don't use artificial sweeteners such as aspartame, saccharin, or acesulfame; however, I do use sucralose (sold as Splenda). The suggestions in the following tables are general guidelines, so the recipes may need some experimentation to achieve desired results.

LIQUID SWEETENERS

SWEETENER	AMOUNT TO USE	WHEN TO USE
Agave Nectar Honey-like liquid from cactus plant. Available in light and dark versions.	1 cup for 1 cup sugar. Reduce liquid ¼ cup per 1 cup agave nectar.	All baked items, puddings, beverages.
Brown Rice Syrup Made from brown rice. Lundberg is gluten free. Half as sweet as sugar.	1⅓ cups for 1 cup sugar. Reduce liquid ¼ cup per each cup of rice syrup. Add ¼ teaspoon baking soda per cup of syrup.	Cookies, pies, puddings. Use with other sweeteners in cakes. Crisps baked goods. Refrigerate after opening.
Corn Syrup Produced by enzymes in cornstarch. Used in many commercial products.	1 cup corn syrup in place of 1 cup white sugar. Reduce liquid by ¼–⅓ cup per cup of syrup.	Any baked item that can use honey.
Frozen Fruit-juice Concentrate (apple, white grape, orange, pineapple). Look for *pure* concentrate.	⅔ cup for 1 cup white sugar. Add ¼ teaspoon baking soda per recipe. Reduce liquid ⅛ cup per each cup of concentrate.	Cakes, cookies, bars. For sweeter flavor, simmer juice on low heat until reduced by ⅓. Cool.
Fruit Puree Use baby food fruits or puree fruits in blender.	Best as substitute for half (not all) sugar or fat. Prune, apple, apricot, banana, and pear are good choices.	Baked goods (e.g., prunes in dark-colored foods, pears in light foods, etc.) The natural pectin in fruits promotes moist, tender baked goods.

SWEETENER	AMOUNT TO USE	WHEN TO USE
Honey From bees. Color and taste depend on flower source. 20–60% sweeter than sugar.	⅔–¾ cup for 1 cup sugar. Reduce liquid ¼ cup per each cup of honey. Add ¼ teaspoon baking soda per cup of honey. Lower oven temperature by 25°F.	All baked goods, beverages, puddings. Don't give honey to children under age two because of possible botulism.
Liquid Fructose Derived from corn.	1 cup liquid fructose in place of 1 cup white sugar. Reduce liquid ¼–⅓ cup per cup of liquid fructose.	Use liquid fructose in same way as honey.
Maple Syrup (Pure) Maple tree sap. Grade B is best in baking. Amber to dark brown in color.	⅔–¾ cup maple syrup for 1 cup white sugar. Reduce liquid by 3 tablespoons per each cup of syrup. Add ⅛ teaspoon baking soda per cup of syrup.	All baked goods, especially cakes. Use organic to avoid formaldehyde and other additives. Refrigerate after opening.
Molasses Concentrated sugar cane juice. Strong flavor.	½ cup molasses for 1 cup white sugar. Reduce liquid by ¼ cup per cup of molasses.	All baked goods. Due to its dark color and dominant flavor, it is best with spiced cakes, muffins, cookies.

Note: Ask your health professional if these alternative sweeteners are safe for your diet.

GRANULAR SWEETENERS

SWEETENER	AMOUNT TO USE	WHEN TO USE
Beet Sugar	1 cup beet sugar for 1 cup white sugar.	In any food that calls for white sugar.
Birch Sugar (Xylitol) From birch trees.	1 cup birch sugar for 1 cup white sugar.	In baked goods, puddings, beverages, and any dish that requires sweetening.
Brown Rice Syrup Powder Made from dried brown rice syrup.	Same amount as sugar. Add ¼ teaspoon baking soda for each cup of brown rice syrup powder.	In puddings, beverages, and all baked goods. Make sure the source is gluten-free. Some brown rice syrup is not gluten free, so the powder may not be, either.
Brown Sugar White sugar with added molasses.	1 cup brown sugar in place of 1 cup white sugar.	Lends heartier flavor and darker color in baked goods. Light and dark versions can be used interchangeably.
Date Sugar Ground, dehydrated dates. Coarse, sweet brown granules.	Use ⅔ as much as sugar. Best used in combination with other sweeteners. Keep dry, cool.	Dissolve in hot liquid first. Burns if baked a long time. Use on fruit desserts. Sift the date granules to filter out larger particles.
Dried Cane Juice (Sucanat, Rapadura) Coarse, amber grains of sugar cane.	Same amount as sugar. Add ¼ teaspoon baking soda per each cup of dried cane juice. Sift before using. Keep dry, cool.	Cookies, cakes, pies, puddings; not white cakes. Dissolve in hot liquid from recipe for less graininess.

SWEETENER	AMOUNT TO USE	WHEN TO USE
FOS (Fructooligo-saccharides) White, low-calorie powder made from fruit.	Half as sweet as sugar.	Best used along with caloric sweeteners in baking, but can be used alone to sweeten cereals, beverages, sauces. May cause gas.
Fructose Powder Usually refined from corn syrup or from fruit sources. Bit sweeter than white sugar.	1 cup fructose powder in place of 1 cup white sugar.	Cakes, cookies, bars, breads, muffins, or any other baked items where sugar is also appropriate. Baked items may brown a bit more quickly.
Granulated Honey Dried honey blended with fructose and maltodextrin.	1 cup granulated honey in place of 1 cup white sugar.	Cookies, cakes, pies, puddings, and any other baked goods where sugar might be used.
Maple Sugar Made from maple syrup boiled down to light-brown granules.	1 cup maple sugar for 1 cup sugar. Add ⅛ teaspoon baking soda for each cup of maple sugar.	Dissolve in hot liquid from recipe before using in batters, if possible. Or sift it to make sure it's fine enough for baking.
Stevia Sweet-leafed herb from Paraguay. Sold as fine, white powder. Contains zero calories.	Pinch. 30 to 40 times sweeter than sugar. Slight licorice aftertaste.	Recipes for baked goods need total revision for best results. Best in beverages, puddings, or nonbaked goods. Contributes none of the browning, moisture, or texture of regular sugar in baking. Use to boost sweetness in a recipe with other sweeteners.

SWEETENER	AMOUNT TO USE	WHEN TO USE
Sucralose (Splenda) Molecule structure of sugar is altered to become noncaloric.	1 cup Splenda in place of 1 cup white sugar.	Beverages, puddings, gelatin, baked goods. Contributes none of the browning, moisture, or texture of regular sugar in baking. Best when combined half and half with sugar or honey.
Turbinado Raw sugar with impurities removed.	1 cup turbinado in place of 1 cup white sugar.	Any recipe, but works better in darker-colored baked goods.

Note: Ask your health professional if these alternative sweeteners are safe for your diet.

FLOUR BLENDS IN BAKING:
MIXES VERSUS INDIVIDUAL INGREDIENTS

Even though you can buy an increasing number of ready-made food items or mixes, the fact remains that (1) you can't buy everything, (2) some of us can't afford to buy lots of ready-made foods, and/or (3) many of us really prefer to prepare our own food from scratch. This means that we still prepare many of our foods at home, rather than ordering them in a restaurant or buying them off the shelf in our local grocery story or health food store.

Many of you have already learned that wheat flour can't be replaced with one single flour in baking. Instead, it takes a blend of flours carefully selected for their unique properties. Measuring all those flours makes baking a bit more time consuming. Isn't there an easier way?

I've pondered the issue of premixed flour blends (several flours blended to measure as one flour) for some time now. Yet, for every customer who wishes I would use flour blends (rather than individually listed ingredients), there are those who are glad I don't, because their food sensitivities don't allow the inflexibility of ready-made blends.

Nonetheless, I—like you—want to minimize my time in the kitchen. For some time now, I have experimented with different blends, using a wide variety of flours. And I've become quite fond of the time-saving convenience of using a flour blend rather than always measuring two, three, or four flours per recipe. This raises the issue of which blend of flours to recommend to you in this book.

I know that some of you can't or don't want to eat legumes (which rules out the bean flours), or you don't like the grittiness of rice flour, or you're allergic to nut flours. So, I devised a flour blend to allow you the most flexibility. It has many variations, so there is sure to be one that suits your taste. The choice is yours about which flours to use in the blend, and you can be assured that every variation works well with the recipes in this book. The only recipes that don't offer you the choice of using my flour blend are those that rely on a specific set of flours to work well, such as the bagels or bread sticks.

This flour blend uses sorghum, which has a pleasingly neutral taste that most seem to like. You have the flexibility of using potato starch, cornstarch, or amaranth starch. You then use tapioca, a pure white flour that has no taste. It is the final half cup of flour, which can include corn, almond, bean, or chestnut, that will give the blend its defining characteristics. See below for more information about how each flour affects the blend.

Regardless of which flours you choose, mix up a large batch and store it on your pantry shelf or in your refrigerator and it will be ready the next time you bake.

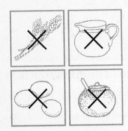

FLOUR BLEND

Makes 4½ cups

1½ cups sorghum flour
1½ cups potato starch, cornstarch, or amaranth starch
1 cup tapioca flour
½ cup corn flour, almond flour, bean flour, or chestnut flour

You can experiment with the variations of this flour blend to see which ones you like best, varying the flours to suit your needs. My favorite blend—the one I use in my personal baking at home—combines sorghum flour, potato starch, tapioca flour, and corn flour (which I grind from white cornmeal). When I want some variety, or the higher protein content from the nut flours, I often use almond flour or chestnut flour. All of the ingredients in this flour blend are readily available at your health food store or possibly your grocery store, but if they're new to you—read on. (To order, see Resources.)

Keep the flour blend in a tightly closed container in a dark, dry place—perhaps your pantry shelf. Unless, of course, you use the nut flours—and then you should refrigerate the flour blend. Bring it to room temperature before using. I like to use widemouthed glass jars because spooning and measuring from them is much easier. Others like to re-cycle the widemouthed plastic containers from Twin Valley Mills that sorghum is packed in (www.twinvalleymills.com). (To order, see Resources.)

Secrets to Success with
Gluten-Free Baking

I still have some mini-disasters in the kitchen, but I've learned a lot of secrets that I share with you in this book. If you follow these general guidelines, your baked goods—cakes, cookies, breads, or anything!—will turn out just fine. You'll find more baking tips specific to bread—an area that I get lots of questions about—in the Breads recipe section (see page 13).

- A combination of gluten-free flours produces a better texture than single flours. For example, brown rice flour—when combined with potato starch and tapioca flour—is far less gritty than brown rice flour used alone. So, always use a blend of flours in your baking.
- Measure flour by stirring it first to aerate it. Place the measuring cup on the counter. Spoon the flour into it, but don't pack it down. Using the straightedge of a knife, level the flour even with the top of the cup. This is the method used in de-veloping all of the recipes in this book.

  If you choose, instead, to dip the measuring cup into the flour and level it off by pressing it against the inside of the bag, you will actually add 1–2 tablespoons more flour per cup than the recipe needs. We call this the "dip and sweep" method of mea-suring, and using it could make your baked goods too dry or ruin them altogether.
- Smaller recipes (those containing 2 cups of flour or less) are easier to adapt to gluten-free flours. Recipes containing cake flour are especially easy to adapt, since they don't depend upon gluten for their structure.

- Gluten-free flours may require more leavening to compensate for their lack of elasticity. As a general rule, if you're converting your own recipes to be gluten free, use about 25 percent more baking soda or baking powder than in the wheat version. However, it usually isn't necessary to increase the yeast in yeast breads.
- If your recipe calls for yeast, dissolve it in the liquid portion of the recipe before adding to the rest of the ingredients. This helps the bread rise better because the yeast will start rising sooner. In some recipes—especially flatbreads that don't have to rise as much—you can just add the yeast along with the dry ingredients.
- Parchment paper or silicone liners are an excellent way to prevent baked goods such as cookies from sticking to the baking sheet.
- Remember that oven temperatures can vary tremendously among different ovens. Buy an oven thermometer and check the temperature of your oven.

STORING YOUR BAKED GOODS

Gluten-free baked goods are usually best warm from the oven. Since home-baked dishes don't have preservatives, their shelf life is short. It's best to refrigerate baked goods to prolong their freshness, but most of us can't eat the entire batch before its shelf life expires.

Many experienced cooks cut the baked items such as bread into individual slices, insert waxed paper between the slices, and freeze them—tightly wrapped. Frozen baked goods, especially breads and muffins, should be thawed gently at room temperature or gently defrosted at 30% power in a microwave oven until thawed. Don't use the microwave's full power to defrost baked goods because it makes them rubbery and tough.

Appendix B

Common Sources of Wheat, Gluten, Dairy, Eggs, Corn & Soy

The following entries are foods or ingredients that are often suspected of including traces of common food allergens. This appendix is based on the latest information from gluten-free and food-allergy experts, but manufacturing practices can change, ingredients can be modified, or new ingredients can be introduced to previously safe foods. So, to put a new slant on an old phrase, it's "*eater* beware." As always, the responsibility for what you eat lies with you. If you have any doubts about a food—*don't eat it!*

Common Sources of Wheat and Gluten

It also important to note that *any* food can be a problem to certain people, regardless of whether they have celiac disease or not. You can have food sensitivities in addition to celiac disease. So, just because you have a reaction to a certain food does not mean that food contains gluten.

This section is based on information from *Gluten-Free Living,* the national magazine for people with gluten sensitivity; the Gluten-Free Living conference by Ann Whelan, September 2003; and the *Quick Start Diet Guide* by the Gluten Intolerance Group and the Celiac Disease Foundation.

BEVERAGES

Distilled liquors—such as scotch, whiskey, and bourbon—do not contain gluten because the gluten peptides cannot survive the distillation process. However, beverages such as beer and ale are fermented rather than distilled and contain gluten from the barley or wheat from which they are made. Wine is made from grapes and does not contain gluten. Unless you know the source of the flavor, beware any alcoholic beverage (even if it is presumed to be safe, such as vodka) if it has flavorings added after distillation. Some hard ciders are gluten-free, since they are made from fermented fruit. Nonalcoholic beverages such as flavored coffees, Postum, and Ovaltine may contain gluten.

BREADS

Unless the label says "gluten-free," avoid biscuits, breads, crackers, croutons, crumbs, doughnuts, tortillas, or wafers. Also, avoid breads made of spelt, kamut, barley, rye, and triticale. Words on the label that indicate wheat include "semolina," "durum," "white flour," "unbleached flour," and "all-purpose flour."

BROWN RICE SYRUP

This can be made from barley; however, Lundberg Brown Rice Syrup is gluten-free.

CANDY

Wheat may be used to prevent sticking during the shaping or handling of candy. Wheat may also be an ingredient in candy, such as licorice, to give it body.

CANOLA OIL

This healthy oil is made from canola seed and is no longer made from rapeseed. It is gluten-free.

CARAMEL COLOR

This *may* contain malt syrup or wheat starch if the product is foreign-made. In the United States, caramel color is most likely made from corn, since corn produces a better product, and the only two manufacturers of caramel color in the United States use corn.

CEREAL

Avoid those made from wheat, rye, barley, spelt, and kamut or cereals that contain malt flavoring or malt syrup. Oats are naturally gluten-free, but may be contaminated with wheat, so it's best to avoid oat cereals as well. There is an increasing array of cereals made from corn, rice, buckwheat, sorghum, quinoa, and amaranth, so you still have plenty of choices.

CITRIC ACID

This is always a suspicious ingredient since citric acid can be fermented from corn, beets, molasses—or wheat. While corn is the only source used by manufacturers in the United States, about 25 percent of the citric acid used in food and drink in the United States is imported from other countries and could contain wheat. By the way, Coke and Pepsi use corn in their citric acid.

COFFEE

Pure coffee is gluten-free, but some flavored coffees may use wheat as a flavor carrier. Make sure that instant coffee is just pure coffee, without wheat as a filler. Labels on coffee substitutes, such as those made from grains, should be read carefully.

CONDIMENTS AND BAKING INGREDIENTS

Wheat-free tamari soy sauce is usually gluten-free. Pure spices are gluten-free, but some spice mixes *may* contain wheat as a filler. Lea & Perrins Worcestershire sauce is gluten-free in the United States, but not in Canada. Coleman's dry mustard contains wheat, so grind your own mustard seeds. Condiments such as ketchup and mustard—which were previously off-limits because of the distilled vinegar—are usually gluten-free unless the label lists a gluten-containing ingredient. Check labels on all condiments to be safe.

DAIRY PRODUCTS

Some flavored or low-fat yogurts contain modified food starch (which is probably corn, but *could* be wheat). Look for the source of the modified food starch on the label. It will most likely be corn, especially if it's made in the United States. Or choose yogurts with pectin (fruit-based). Malted milk, processed cheese spread, low-fat sour cream, and chocolate milk *may* contain wheat.

Desserts and Other Sweets

Avoid commercial pudding mixes, some cake decorations, and marzipan. Look for the words "gluten-free" on the label of commercially baked goods.

Dextrin

In the United States, it is usually made from corn or tapioca. But it can be made from wheat, so avoid this ingredient.

Distilled Vinegar

Experts believe that gluten cannot survive the distillation process, so grain-based vinegars (except malt vinegar) are considered gluten-free. (See *Gluten-Free Living* magazine, Vol. 8, #3.) Malt vinegar has malt flavor from barley added in *after* distillation, so it is not gluten-free. If flavorings or seasonings are added to the vinegar after distillation, check the label for ingredients. Wine, rice, and cider vinegar are still good choices for the gluten-free diet.

Flavorings

Generally speaking, natural flavorings are gluten-free. However, natural flavorings used in or on meats *may* contain gluten, since wheat has a natural affinity for meat and meat products.

Grains

The "new" grains such as amaranth, buckwheat, sorghum, quinoa, and teff are gluten-free. In most cases, these grains are not even botanically related to wheat.

Hydrolyzed Vegetable Protein

The word "vegetable" can mean anything. However, since 1993, this ingredient can't appear on a food label. But it may still be possible to find old foods that still bear this ingredient. Today, the ingredient would be labeled with its source, such as "hydrolyzed soy protein."

MALT
Malt is made from barley and therefore contains gluten.

MALTODEXTRIN
In the United States, maltodextrin cannot legally be made from gluten but is made from corn, rice, or potato. So, unless your product is foreign made, the maltodextrin should not contain gluten.

MEAT, FISH, AND EGGS
Avoid any meat that's been breaded or in which fillers might be used, such as sausage, luncheon meats, or hot dogs. Avoid self-basting turkeys. Buy tuna in spring water rather than oil. Egg substitutes are not necessarily pure eggs and contain many additional ingredients, such as wheat.

MODIFIED FOOD STARCH
It is usually corn when used in food but could be wheat or some other food starch, especially when made outside the United States. The content of the modified food starch should be declared on the label. The word "starch" usually means cornstarch. However, when starch is used in pharmaceuticals, these rules may not apply.

MONO- AND DIGLYCERIDES
These are fats and not a concern in their liquid state. If they are used in their dry form, then wheat might be used. However, wheat is declared on the label by two major food manufacturers, Kraft and General Mills.

PASTAS
Look for "gluten-free" on the label. You can eat Oriental rice noodles, bean threads, and commercial pasta made from pure buckwheat or those made from beans, corn, quinoa, potato starch, or rice.

SEASONINGS

These are usually made from combinations of herbs and spices and may have a carrier such as wheat flour, which may or may not be declared.

SOUPS AND CHOWDERS

Many canned soups, soup mixes, and bouillon cubes or granules contain wheat as a thickener or filler.

SOY SAUCE

Always look for wheat-free tamari soy sauce, because regular soy sauce is made with wheat.

SPICES

A pure spice that only has one name (e.g., cinnamon) is made from cinnamon only. If there is no ingredient label, then the cinnamon is pure cinnamon with no additives or fillers. Pure spices (those with just one spice or herb) are usually gluten-free, especially the McCormick brand.

TEXTURED VEGETABLE PROTEIN

This ingredient is usually made from soy, not wheat.

VANILLA

Vanilla is now known to be gluten-free because gluten cannot survive the distillation process. If in doubt, look for gluten-free, nonalcohol flavorings.

VEGETABLES

"Vegetable starch" or "vegetable protein" on the label could mean corn, peanuts, rice, soy, or wheat. Avoid vegetables that are breaded, creamed, or scalloped.

Yeast

Baker's yeast used in breads is gluten-free. Common brands such as Red Star and Fleischmann's are gluten-free. Nutritional yeast (a supplement) and brewer's yeast (a by-product of the brewing industry) may or may not be gluten-free, so check with the manufacturer. Autolyzed yeast, commonly used as a food flavoring, is generally gluten-free.

To stay informed about ingredient safety, subscribe to *Gluten-Free Living* magazine, or visit Web sites such as www.celiac.com and www.clanthompson.com. Or purchase the Commercial Product Listing from the Celiac Sprue Association or the product listing from the Tri-County Celiac Support Group. See Resources for addresses.

COMMON SOURCES OF DAIRY

Milk and milk products are hidden in many foods. Your food choices should be guided by whether you are lactose-intolerant or allergic to milk proteins. Many words indicate milk—casein is a milk protein; whey, another protein, is the liquid derived from drained yogurt. Other terms to avoid are: "acidophilus," "caseinate," "calcium caseinate," "hydrolyzed milk protein" or "vegetable protein," "lactalbumin," "lactate," "lactoglobulin," "lactose," and "potassium caseinate." Below is a partial list of hidden dairy sources.

Baked Goods/Cooking Ingredients
Biscuits
Bread
Cakes
Caramel coloring or flavoring
Chocolate
Cookies
Doughnuts
Hotcakes
Malted milk
Mixes for cakes, cookies, doughnuts, muffins, pancakes, etc.

Ovaltine (and other cocoa drinks)
Pie crust (made with milk products)
Soda crackers
Zwieback

Casseroles/Side Dishes
Creamed vegetables
Dishes in au gratin style
Fritters
Hash
Mashed potatoes
Rarebit
Scalloped dishes

Dairy
Buttermilk
Cheese
Condensed milk
Cream
Cream cheese
Evaporated milk
Ghee (clarified butter)
Ice cream
Milk (all forms)
Nondairy creamer
Skim milk powder
Sour cream
Whey
Yogurt

Desserts
Bavarian cream
Candies
Custard
Ice cream, sherbet, and
    gelato
Pudding
Sorbet (some versions)
Spumoni

Egg Dishes
Omelets
Scrambled eggs
Soufflé

Meats/Fish
Canned tuna
Deli turkey
Hamburger
Meat fried in butter
Sausage

Pharmaceuticals
Lactose is often used
    as a filler.

Sauces/Salad Dressings
Butter sauce
Cream sauce
Gravy

Hard sauce
Mayonnaise (some brands)
Salad dressing (some)

Soups
Bisque
Chowder

COMMON SOURCES OF EGGS

Many commercially prepared foods—or ingredients used to prepare your own dishes—contain eggs. Here is a partial list of those items. Be sure to read labels and remember that the ingredient list may not specifically mention the word "eggs," but instead use words such as "albumen," "livetin," "ovaglubin egg albumen," "ovamucin," "ovumucoid," "ovovitellin," "lysozyme," or "egg whites," "egg yolks," "egg solids," or "egg powder."

Baked Goods/Cooking
    Ingredients
Baking powder
Batter for deep frying
Bread
Breaded food
Cake
Cake flour
Cinnamon rolls
Cookies
Doughnuts
French toast

Fritters
Frosting
Icing
Malted cocoa drinks
Marshmallows
Muffins
Pancake flour
Pancake mixes
Pancakes
Pretzels
Waffle mixes
Waffles

Beverages
Eggnog
Malted cocoa drinks
    (e.g., Ovaltine)
Wine (may be "cleared" with
    egg whites)

Condiments/Sauces
Hollandaise sauce
Salad dressing (especially
    boiled ones)

Sauce (may be thickened
with eggs)
Tartar sauce

Desserts
Bavarian cream
Ice cream
Ices
Macaroons
Meringues
Pie (cream pie filling and
some pie crusts)

Pudding
Sherbet
Soufflé

*Meats/Meat-related
Dishes*
Bouillon
Hamburger mix
Meatballs
Meat jellies
Meat loaf
Meat molds

Pâté (also called foie gras)
Patties
Sausage
Soup (e.g., consommé)
Spaghetti and meatballs

Other
Pasta (and dishes containing
pasta)
Tartar sauce

COMMON SOURCES OF CORN

Corn appears in many unsuspecting places as an emulsifier, sweetener, or main
ingredient.

*Baked Goods/Cooking
Ingredients*
Baking mixes for biscuits,
doughnuts, pancakes, and
pies
Baking powder
Batters and deep-frying
mixtures
Bleached wheat flour
Breads and pastries
Cakes
Cereals
Cookies
Corn syrup
Cream pies
Glucose products
Graham crackers
Oleo or margarine
Powdered sugar

Tortillas
Vanilla extract
Vinegar (distilled)
Xanthan gum

Beverages
Ales and beer
Bourbon
Carbonated beverages
Fruit juices
Grape juice (look for pure
grape juice)
Instant coffee
Milk (in paper cartons)
Soy milk
Tea (instant)
Whiskey
Wines (some contain corn)

*Condiments/Sauces/
Snacks*
Cheese
Commercial syrups
(e.g., Karo)
Fritos, tortilla chips
Ketchup
Peanut butter
Popcorn
Salad dressings (e.g., French)
Soups (cream-style)

Desserts
Candy
Frosting
Gelatin or Jell-O
Ice cream
Jams, jellies
Puddings and custards

Sauces for cakes or sundaes
Sherbet

Meats/Side Dishes
Bacon
Bologna
Canned peas
Chili
Chop suey
Gravy, sauce for meats
Grits
Ham
Sandwich spread
Sausage
Vegetables (in cream sauces)

Nonfood Items
Adhesives and glue
Bath powder
Envelopes, stamps
Plastic food wrappers
Talcum powder
Toothpaste

*Pharmaceuticals/Drugs/
    Additives*
Aspirin, cough syrup, and
    other tablets
Dextrin, dextrose
Mannitol

MSG (monosodium
    glutamate)
NutraSweet, Splenda
Sorbitol
Vitamin C preparations

COMMON SOURCES OF SOY

Soy appears in many commercially prepared foods as well as in many ingredients.

*Baked Goods/Cooking
    Ingredients*
Breads
Cakes
Cereals
Cooking spray
Crackers
Lecithin (derived from soy)
Oils
Oleo or margarine
Pastries
Rolls
Shortening

Beverages
Coffee substitutes
Lemonade mix
Soy milk

*Condiments/Sauces/
    Snacks/Soups*
Butter substitute
Cheese
Salad dressing
Soup
Soy sauce (and other Orien-
    tal sauces)
Worcestershire sauce

Desserts
Candy
Candy bars
Caramel
Custard
Ice cream
Nut candies

*Meats/Meat-related
    Dishes*
Luncheon meats
Sausage (certain kinds)

Miscellaneous
Baby foods
Bean sprouts
Pasta from soy flour
Tempura
Tofu

Appendix C

CONVERTING BUTTER OR MARGARINE TO OIL

If you want to use oil instead of butter or margarine, the chart below tells you how much to use. Amounts are approximate and may vary across recipes.

Butter/Margarine Oil	Oil
1 teaspoon	¾ teaspoon
1 tablespoon	2¼ teaspoons
2 tablespoons	1½ tablespoons
¼ cup	3 tablespoons
⅓ cup	¼ cup
½ cup	¼ cup + 2 tablespoons
⅔ cup	½ cup
¾ cup	½ cup + 1 tablespoon
1 cup	¾ cup

Appendix D

Food Measures & Equivalents

This handy chart shows food measures and equivalents.

AMOUNT	MEASURE
Berries	
1 pint	2¾ cups
Butter/Margarine	
1 pound	4 sticks/2 cups
1 stick	½ cup (8 tablespoons)
Cheese	
8 ounces cottage cheese	1 cup
8 ounces cream cheese	1 cup
4 ounces Parmesan	1¼ cups

AMOUNT	MEASURE
Chocolate	
1 square	4 tablespoons cocoa
1 square	3 tablespoons cocoa +1 tablespoon oil
Cream	
1 cup heavy cream	2 cups whipped
Dried Beans/Peas	
1 cup	2¼ cups cooked

AMOUNT	MEASURE
Flour	
1 pound	4 cups
Herbs	
1 tablespoon fresh	1 teaspoon dried
Pasta	
8 ounces angel-hair	5½ cups cooked
8 ounces elbow	4 cups cooked
8 ounces noodles	3¾ cups cooked
8 ounces spaghetti	4 cups cooked

AMOUNT	MEASURE
Rice	
1 cup brown	3–4 cups cooked
1 cup instant	1½ cups cooked
1 cup white	3 cups cooked
Sugar	
1 pound brown	2¼ cups
1 pound granulated	2 cups
1 pound powdered	4½ cups

Appendix E

APPLIANCES, PANS & UTENSILS

Appliances

People often ask me what type of appliances I use when developing recipes for my cookbooks. I use Breadman, Welbilt, and Zojirushi bread machines. When mixing large recipes or heavy bread dough by hand, I use a 4.5-quart KitchenAid stand mixer with regular beaters—not dough hooks.

For cake, cookie batters, and cooking class demonstrations, I use a handheld Hamilton Beach mixer. My KitchenAid food processor, fitted with the knife blade, is fabulous for blending dough. It is fast and does a better job of distributing the moisture throughout the ingredients than an electric mixer. In fact, I wouldn't be without this indispensable appliance (less expensive versions are $40 at discount stores).

My range is an electric Jenn-Air, and I have two ovens: an electric Jenn-Air and an electric KitchenAid. Remember that different brands and types of ovens may produce slightly different outcomes. For example, in my experience gas ovens can be a little hotter. It's best to follow the directions exactly the first time you make any recipe; then make changes as needed—such as longer or shorter baking times.

I love my small, handheld coffee grinder. About $10, it grinds mustard seeds into mustard powder perfectly. To clean the coffee grinder, pulverize a tablespoon of white rice kernels, discard the rice, and wipe the interior of the grinder with damp paper towels to clean it. Avoid using the same grinder for grinding coffee or else your mustard or other spices will taste like coffee. I use a microplane zester, available at cooking stores, to grate lemon peel.

PANS

I bake almost exclusively in gray nonstick pans to keep gluten-free batters from sticking. Also, their gray finish (rather than shiny aluminum) helps the browning process. Black nonstick pans tend to burn gluten-free batters. Insulated baking pans tend to make baked goods somewhat soggy (except for some cookies). Be sure to use utensils that won't scratch the nonstick surface of the pan. It is better to bake in several smaller pans instead of one large pan so that the finished product will rise and bake more evenly and thoroughly.

PAN SUBSTITUTIONS

When choosing pan sizes, measure across top of pan, from inside edge to inside edge. For fluted baking molds, measure from inside edge of outward curve to inside of exact opposite curve. Measure depth on inside vertical from bottom of dish or pan to top edge. To determine volume of pan or dish, fill with water. Then, pour water into measuring cup.

PAN OR DISH	EQUIVALENT IN CUPS
13x9-inch baking pan	12–15 cups
10x4-inch tube pan	12 cups
10x3½-inch Bundt pan	12 cups
9x3-inch tube pan	9 cups
9x3-inch Bundt pan	9 cups
11x7-inch baking pan	8 cups
8-inch square baking pan	8 cups
9x5-inch loaf pan	8 cups

9-inch deep-dish pie plate	6–8 cups
9x1½-inch cake pan	6 cups
7½x3-inch Bundt pan	6 cups
9x1½-inch cake pan	5 cups
8x1½-inch cake pan	4–5 cups
8x4-inch loaf pan	4 cups

Here are the most common sizes for various pots and pans.

Dutch Ovens	Shallow Baking Dishes
Small = 2 quart	Small = 1 quart
Medium = 6 quart	Medium = 2 quart
Large = 8 quart	Large = 3 quart
Roasting Pans	**Skillets**
Small = 13x9x2 inches	Small = 7- or 8-inch diameter
Medium = 14x11x2 inches	Medium = 9- or 10-inch diameter
Large = 16x13x3 inches	Large = 11- or 12-inch diameter
Saucepans	**Stockpots**
Small = 1 quart	Small = 6–8 quart
Medium = 1½–2 quart	Medium = 12 quart
Large = 4 quart	Large = 16–20 quart

Utensils & Other Helpers

Use serrated knives or electric knives for cutting breads or pie crust. Use waxed paper or parchment paper for baked goods that must be removed from the pan whole, rather than sliced. Use heavy-duty plastic wrap for making pie crust.

Glossary of Ingredients

Read this section carefully so you know what the ingredient is, what it looks like, and where to find it (if it is not available in grocery stores). No endorsement of products is intended, but I mention certain brands to help you find the ingredient in the United States, although product brands vary by region. The information in this section applies to the United States only, not to foods or ingredients manufactured outside the United States.

Read labels carefully to make sure you know what is in the food. Continue to read labels since manufacturers can change the ingredients and the processes under which the ingredient is handled. And remember . . . *if in doubt about any ingredient, don't eat it!*

Agave Nectar: A honey-like liquid made from the agave plant, this sweetener is 90 percent fructose. Found in baking aisle of health food stores and increasingly in grocery stores near the honey. See Baking with Alternative Sweeteners in Appendix A for guidelines on using it in baking.

Applesauce: Also available as baby food, but choose those (e.g., Gerber First) that don't contain extra fillers, such as rice or tapioca. Organic versions are usually darker and will cause baked goods to be somewhat darker. See Baking Without Conventional Ingredients in Appendix A for guidelines on using it.

Amaranth: A super-nutritious grain, originally grown by the Aztecs. See Baking Without Conventional Ingredients in Appendix A for guidelines on using it. Available from www.nuworldamaranth.com. Amaranth starch is the starch from the seed and does not contain the same nutrient profile as the whole seed.

Arrowroot: White powder made from a West Indies root. It is an excellent thickener for fruit sauces or other sauces that do not require high heat. It can also be used as a flour in baking. Binds baked goods. Found in health food stores. See Baking Without Conventional Ingredients in Appendix A for guidelines on using it.

Ascorbic Acid: Also called Vitamin C crystals or powder. Choose unbuffered version for maximum leavening boost in baked goods. Found in supplements at health food stores. (See **Vitamin C Crystals or Powder.**)

Baking Powder: Ener-G and Featherweight brands make grain-free versions. Despite concerns over baking powder, I have yet to find a brand that contains wheat.

Birch Sugar: Also known as xylitol, this white sugar comes from the birch tree and measures just like white sugar. Found in the health food store, although it is costly and somewhat hard to find.

Brown Rice Syrup: Made from brown rice. Lundberg's brand is gluten-free. Found in health food stores.

Brown Sugar: Generally made from cane sugar, this is white refined sugar to which a little molasses has been added. It comes in light and dark versions, although most recipes in this book use the light version.

Butter: If cow's-milk butter is unsuitable, use margarine or use canola oil spread (Spectrum or Earth Balance or Soy Garden), vegetable shortening, or the same amount of your favorite cooking oil (may need to reduce the amount of oil). (See also **Buttery Spread** and **Oil** below.)

Butter-Flavored Salt or **Sprinkles:** Durkee makes a gluten-free version and Butter Buds are gluten-free, but both may be derived from dairy. Instead, use the same amount of butter-flavored extract.

Buttery Spread: This is the term applied to nondairy, nonhydrogenated spreads that look and taste like butter. It is made from different blends of oils including canola, palm, and soy, by brands such as Earth Balance, Soy Garden, and Spectrum. They bake quite well, but some versions (e.g., canola oil spread by Spectrum) do not melt or blend into sauces cooked on the stove. The fat is mostly monounsaturated, so they are a healthy substitute for vegetable shortening, margarine, or butter—which you may use instead. Found in refrigerated section near the butter in health food stores and some supermarkets.

Canola Oil: One of the most heart-healthy oils, it has a very low smoking point, so it won't cause baked goods to brown too quickly. You may substitute other oils, such as safflower, corn, or vegetable.

Cheese: See **Parmesan Cheese** below and also see Baking Without Conventional Ingredients in Appendix A for more information on related dairy products.

Chipotle Chiles: Dried jalapeño peppers. Found in Mexican section in supermarket or health food store. Chipotles in adobo sauce may contain wheat flour as a thickener.

Chocolate and **Chocolate Chips:** Gluten-free, dairy-free chocolates are made by Tropical Source and usually found in health food stores. Chocolate that is free of gluten and dairy is also available at www.enjoylifefoods.com, www.ener-g.com, www.kirkman-labs.com, www.allergygrocer.com, www.soyfreechocolateco.com, and www.choclat.com. Some brands of dairy-free chocolate chips and bars are available in health food stores, but may actually be processed on dairy equipment. Carob chips may be used instead of chocolate chips, but they may have been sweetened with barley malt, which contains gluten. Read the labels carefully on all chocolates, especially those that are flavored, to make sure their ingredients are safe for you.

Cocoa Powder: Use unsweetened cocoa powder, unless the recipe says otherwise. Carob powder may be used, but with a significant loss of flavor and color.

Coffee Powder: Sanka and Maxim make gluten-free instant coffee powder. Espresso powder (Medaglia D'Oro) may be used instead.

Cooking Spray: Put your favorite oil in a nonaerosol pump-spray bottle, available at kitchen stores. I prefer to use vegetable shortening to grease baking pans instead of cooking spray.

Corn Flour: Made from the whole corn kernel and used in baking or breading mixes. Grind your own from gluten-free cornmeal, or buy in the health food store. Shiloh Farms (see Resources) offers a gluten-free version. See Baking Without Conventional Ingredients in Appendix A for guidelines on using it.

Cornstarch: Made from corn, this white powder is the same ingredient used to thicken sauces and puddings. Can be used as a flour in wheat-free cooking, but it is not the same as corn flour (which is ground from the whole corn kernel, is yellow, and has a heavier texture). See Baking Without Conventional Ingredients in Appendix A for guidelines on using it.

Dry Milk Powder: This fine, white milk powder adds sugar and protein to baked goods. Better Than Milk, Solait, English Bay Dairy-Free, and Vance's DariFree are nondairy substitutes. Found in health food stores. Carnation instant milk doesn't measure the same as dry milk powder, so use twice as much.

Egg Replacer Powder: White powder made of various starches and leavening. Use in addition to eggs in certain recipes or in place of eggs in others. Helps stabilize baked goods. Ener-G or Kingsmill brands are sold in health food stores. See Baking Without Conventional Ingredients in Appendix A.

Eggs: Use large eggs, which equal about ¼ cup each. See Baking with Egg Substitutes in Appendix A.

Flaxseed or **Flaxseed Meal:** Seeds or meal (partially ground seeds) are used as an egg substitute. Found in health food stores. See Baking Without Conventional Ingredients in Appendix A.

Garlic Powder or **Garlic Salt:** Durkee and Spice Islands are gluten-free. Or use fresh garlic instead and alter the amount of salt as needed.

Gelatin Powder: Available in regular version (common brand name is Knox or Grayslake) or kosher, which is made from vegetable sources. It adds moisture and helps bind ingredients together. Kosher versions are at some health food stores and may be marked "pareve." Or buy ClearJel from King Arthur Flour catalog (at www.bakerscatalogue.com).

Guar Gum: Plant-derived gum used to provide structure to baked goods so leavening can do its job. It contains fiber, so it could irritate the digestive tract if used in large amounts. Can be used in place of xanthan gum, but use half again as much guar gum. Found in baking aisle of health food stores or from online gluten-free vendors (see Mail-Order Sources).

Italian Seasoning: A blend of spices and herbs, found in the spice section of the baking aisle of grocery stores and health food stores. It is not the seasoning packets used to make salad dressings.

Lecithin Granules: Made from soy, lecithin emulsifies, stabilizes, and texturizes baked goods (especially bread). Found in the supplement department of health food stores (sometimes in the refrigerated sections). Usually light or yellow-beige in color, the limited amount required (about ¼ teaspoon) does not change the flavor or appearance of the dish but does produce a finer texture in baking and makes other dishes seem richer, as though they had more fat. Buy only *pure* soy lecithin.

Lemon Zest (Peel or **Rind):** Outermost portion of the lemon; does not include the yellow pith under it. Adds flavor to baked goods. Use a microplane grater or zester to remove zest from lemon. Use organic produce to avoid pesticides.

Maple Syrup: Made from maple tree sap and available at supermarkets and health food stores. Most flavorful version for baking is Grade B, which is often sold in bulk in health food stores. Choose organic maple syrup to avoid formaldehyde. See Baking Without Conventional Ingredients in Appendix A for guidelines on using maple syrup.

Margarine: Can be used in place of butter, but diet margarines have too much water for use in baking. Nonhydrogenated brands—called buttery spreads—are made by Earth Balance, Soy Garden, and Spectrum and are found in health food stores. See Baking Without Conventional Ingredients in Appendix A for guidelines on using it.

Milk: People with dairy allergies or lactose intolerance should use alternatives such as rice, soy, potato, or nut milks (called "beverages"). Choose casein-free substitutes if you're allergic to dairy, or lactose-free products if you're lactose intolerant. The Food Allergy & Anaphylaxis Network (FAAN) (www.foodallergy.org) forbids goat milk for dairy-allergic and lactose-intolerant people. Check with your physician.

People with celiac disease should avoid milk substitutes that contain barley malt or oats because these ingredients contain gluten. Read labels to choose one appropriate for your condition. Use low-sugar or unsweetened milks for savory dishes. See Baking Without Conventional Ingredients in Appendix A for guidelines on using nondairy products.

Millet: An often neglected grain in the gluten-free diet yet a highly nutritious alternative to wheat. See Baking Without Conventional Ingredients in Appendix A for guidelines on using it.

Molasses: Use regular (unsulphured) molasses, not blackstrap molasses, which is far stronger in flavor. See Baking Without Conventional Ingredients in Appendix A for guidelines on using molasses.

Montina: A flour ground from Indian rice grass which is cultivated in Montana (hence the name). Very high in fiber and protein, it is sold as a pure supplement or blended with rice flour and tapioca flour. See Baking Without Conventional Ingredients in Appendix A for guidelines on using it.

Mustard: For dry mustard powder, choose Durkee or Spice Islands. Or grind mustard seeds to a fine powder in a small spice or coffee grinder. Coleman's, a popular brand, contains gluten. For prepared mustards, the original concern was vinegar. We now know that, unless it is malt vinegar, it is gluten-free and most likely corn-based. Even if it was made with wheat-based vinegar, the gluten peptides could not survive the distillation process. For more information on vinegar, see *Gluten-Free Living* magazine (Vol. 8, #3, 2003) or the brochure "Is Vinegar Safe for Celiacs?" © 2002. Available from www.glutenfreeliving.com.

Nut Milk: Nondairy beverages made from almonds or hazelnuts. Read the labels to make sure the other ingredients are safe for your diet. Nut milks are sold in health food stores. You can make your own nut milk with recipes from this book.

Oil: The heart-healthiest oils are canola and olive oil. Safflower, canola, and corn oils work well in baking due to their low smoking points. (See **Canola Oil** and **Safflower Oil**.)

Onion Powder, Onion Salt, and **Dried Minced Onion:** Look for gluten-free versions by Durkee or Spice Islands or use freshly grated onion and adjust the salt accordingly when replacing onion salt.

Parmesan Cheese: This cheese made from cow's milk comes in either a grated or shredded version or in hard chunks that you grate or shred yourself. Soyco makes a brown rice version that contains casein (a milk protein) and another version made of soy, labeled 100 percent dairy free and casein free. Store on pantry shelf until opened, then refrigerate.

Potato Flour: A heavy, slightly off-white flour made from the whole potato (including the skin). It is used in very small amounts and lends some "chew" and weight to baked goods. It also has a much stronger flavor than the relatively neutral-flavored potato starch. Found in the flour section of health food stores. See Baking Without Conventional Ingredients in Appendix A for guidelines on using it.

Potato Starch: Also called potato starch flour. Fine, white powder made from the starch of potatoes. It adds a light, airy texture to baked goods and also makes an excellent thickener. Found in the flour section of health food stores. Don't confuse it with the heavy, dense potato flour made from whole potatoes (including their skins). See Baking Without Conventional Ingredients in Appendix A for guidelines on using it.

Pureed Fruit: Several fruits work nicely to help bind ingredients, add sweetness and moisture, and replace fat due to their natural pectins and natural sugars. Pureed pears impart little flavor or color. Pureed apples (applesauce or apple butter) impart a slight apple flavor, especially if the apple butter is spiced. The darker color and flavor of pureed prunes or dates make them useful only in darker, more strongly flavored dishes such as spice cakes or chocolate items. See Baking Without Conventional Ingredients in Appendix A for guidelines.

Quinoa: This ancient, highly nutritious grain was once grown by the Incas in Peru. The whole grains can be cooked into a hot cereal or side dish, while quinoa flour can be used in baking. See Baking Without Conventional Ingredients in Appendix A for guidelines on using it.

Rice Bran: This is the outside layer of the rice kernel, which is removed to make brown rice. It contains bran and part of the rice germ. Made by Ener-G and sold in the baking aisle of health food stores, near the flours or in the baking aisle. It adds fiber to baked goods. Refrigerate after opening.

Rice Flakes: Closely resembling rolled oats, these are also called rolled rice or rolled rice flakes. Found in health food stores or www.enjoylifefoods.com or www.vitamincottage.com.

Rice Flour: This is the most common flour used in gluten-free baking. White rice flour is the rice kernel stripped of most of its nutrients. Brown rice flour contains more layers of the rice kernel—and more nutrients in comparison to white rice flour. Store brown rice flour in the refrigerator or freezer to extend shelf life and avoid rancidity. Found in baking aisle or bulk sections of health food stores and some supermarkets. See Baking Without Conventional Ingredients in Appendix A for guidelines on using it.

Rice Milk: Also called rice beverage. Made from rice, this milk is an effective substitute for cow's milk. It is available at health food stores or supermarkets. Refrigerate after opening. Choose enriched or fortified versions. Celiacs must avoid those with barley-based brown rice syrup such as Rice Dream or malted cereal extract, which may contain barley. See Baking Without Conventional Ingredients in Appendix A.

Rice Polish: The portion of brown rice kernel removed in the process of making white rice. It contains part of the rice germ and bran—high in fiber, but not as high as rice bran. Refrigerate after opening. Made by Ener-G and sold in the baking aisles of health food stores.

Rolled Rice: See **Rice Flakes.**

Safflower Oil: Made from the safflower plant, this oil works well in baking or sautéing because of its relatively high smoking point, which means that it won't burn as quickly.

Salt: Use your favorite salt, but check the fillers that make them free flowing. I prefer sea salt because it has no fillers—but it is more expensive. You may reduce the salt in recipes to suit your individual taste and dietary needs. However, the overall flavor will be affected since salt is a flavor enhancer.

Sorghum Flour: Once known as milo, this light-beige flour is called white sorghum and comes from the white sorghum plant. Brands by Authentic Foods, Bob's Red Mill Natural Foods, and Ener-G Foods are available in the baking aisle at health food stores. See Baking Without Conventional Ingredients in Appendix A for guidelines.

Sorghum Syrup: A dark-colored syrup, somewhat thicker and heavier than corn syrup, made from a sorghum plant. It can be found in health food stores near the honey or agave nectar.

Sour Cream Alternative: Made from soy and many other ingredients; it performs similar to real sour cream. Found in the dairy section of health food stores. Some brands contain casein or other problematic ingredients, so read labels carefully.

Soy Flour: Derived from soy beans, this yellowish-tan flour is found in regular and lower-fat form—usually in the flour section of health food stores. Refrigerate to avoid rancidity due to fat content. Works best in baked goods with fruit such as carrot cakes. Persons who are allergic to legumes should avoid this flour. See Baking Without Conventional Ingredients in Appendix A for guidelines.

Soy Milk: Also called soy beverage, it is available at health food stores or supermarkets. Refrigerate after opening. Read labels to avoid problem ingredients. See Baking Without Conventional Ingredients in Appendix A for guidelines.

Soy Sauce: Look for the wheat-free tamari version by San-J. You may also use Bragg's Amino Acids, which is a nonfermented soy sauce without wheat or yeast.

Sugar: Bleached or unbleached cane sugar may be used. Beet sugar may also be used. See Baking Without Conventional Ingredients in Appendix A for guidelines.

Sun-dried Tomatoes: Dehydrated tomatoes that are packaged dry or packed in oil. Choose dry packaged version if you prefer a lower fat content.

Sweet Rice Flour: Derived from short-grain rice, this white powder produces baked goods that are more moist and firm than if "long-grain" rice flour is used. Sometimes called "sticky" or "glutinous" rice, it *does not* contain wheat gluten. It is sold in boxes by Ener-G or bags by Bob's Red Mill Natural Foods in the baking aisle in health food stores. See Baking Without Conventional Ingredients in Appendix A.

Tapioca Flour: Made from the cassava plant, this is a fine, white flour that adds chewiness and elasticity to baked goods. It is sold in health food stores in package or bulk form. See Baking Without Conventional Ingredients in Appendix A.

Teff: This is a tiny grain, originally grown in Ethiopia and now provides a nutritious alternative to wheat. It can be cooked as hot cereal or used as flour in baking. See Baking Without Conventional Ingredients in Appendix A for guidelines.

Tofu: Be sure to use the soft silken version made by Mori-Nu in baked goods unless otherwise specified. Store the aseptic (shelf-stable) packages on pantry shelf until opened. Refrigerate in closed container and use within two days. Found in health food stores in refrigerated section or in displays near the baking aisle.

Vanilla Extract: Vanilla is safe for the gluten-free diet. The original concern was the source of the alcohol, but—like vinegar—it is usually made from corn. Even if it was made from wheat, the gluten peptides could not survive the distillation process.

Vegetable Oil: The best oils for baking are canola, safflower, and sunflower because of their higher smoking points, which means they won't burn as quickly. Canola oil is one of the more heart-healthy oils, but you may use your favorite oil. Avoid using olive oil in baking unless specified in the recipe. Most oils are found in baking aisle of supermarkets and health food stores.

Vinegar: Except for malt vinegar, vinegar is gluten-free and most likely corn-based. Even if it was made with wheat, the gluten peptides could not survive the distillation process. For more information on vinegar, see *Gluten-Free Living* magazine (Vol. 8, #3, 2003) or the brochure "Is Vinegar Safe for Celiacs?" © 2002. Available from www.glutenfreeliving.com.

Vitamin C Crystals or **Powder:** Derived from the fermentation of corn, this acidic powder provides food for the yeast in bread dough and strengthens the protein structure. It also acts as an acidic leavening component in quick breads, which are baked in the oven, not in a bread machine. It is sold in the supplement section of health food stores. Make sure the label says "wheat-free" and "gluten-free." Choose unbuffered vitamin C, or it will not add acid to the bread.

Water: Some cooks prefer to use filtered water instead of tap water because it produces a sweeter, fuller flavor in baked goods. And some cooks believe that the chlorine in tap water interferes with the action of the yeast in bread.

Worcestershire Sauce: Lea & Perrins and French's are gluten-free when made in the United States. However, Lea & Perrins made in Canada contains malt vinegar.

Xanthan Gum: Derived from bacteria in corn sugar, this gum lends structure and texture to baked goods and thickens sauces. It is probably the most indispensable ingredient when baking without wheat or gluten. Found in baking aisle or near flours in health food stores. Seems expensive, but lasts a long time since only a tiny amount is used in recipes. Can be used interchangeably with guar gum, but use half again as much guar gum as xanthan gum.

Yeast: Red Star and SAF are gluten-free. In this book, "active dry yeast" is the term used to indicate regular yeast.

Yogurt: Choose yogurts with good acidophilus content. Lactose-reduced yogurt is a possible solution for the lactose intolerant, but check with your physician. Goat's-milk yogurt is not a good solution for either the milk-allergic or lactose-intolerant person, according to the Food Allergy & Anaphylaxis Network (FAAN) (www.foodallergy.org). Soy yogurt is a good substitute for cow's-milk yogurt, but it does not work well in baking. See Baking Without Conventional Ingredients in Appendix A for guidelines.

Note: Much of what we know about which ingredients are safe and which are not is due to the diligent research by *Gluten-Free Living* magazine (www.glutenfreeliving.com). In fact, much of what we've learned from this magazine falls into what we consider "common knowledge," and we forget to give credit where credit is due.

RESOURCES

ASSOCIATIONS FOR THOSE ON SPECIAL DIETS

Ask your physician about local support groups for people with food allergies, celiac disease, or other conditions where certain ingredients must be omitted from one's diet.

ALLERGY & ASTHMA NETWORK,
MOTHERS OF ASTHMATICS, INC.
3554 Chain Ridge Road, Suite 200
Fairfax, VA 22030-2709
(800) 878-4403 (help line);
(703) 385-4403

AMERICAN ACADEMY OF ALLERGY,
ASTHMA & IMMUNOLOGY
611 E. Wells Street
Milwaukee, WI 53202
(800) 822-2762 (help line);
(414) 272-6071

AMERICAN CELIAC SOCIETY DIETARY
SUPPORT COALITION
P.O. Box 23455
New Orleans, LA 70183
www.amerceliacsoc@netscape.net

AMERICAN CELIAC TASK FORCE
www.celiaccenter.org/taskforce.asp
e-mail: actfe-mail: actffogworks.net
For e-mail updates, type "subscribe"
in subject line at:
celiac_list@capwiz.mailmanager.net

AMERICAN DIABETES, INC.
1660 Duke Street
Alexandria, VA 22314
(800) DIABETES or (800) 232-3472
www.diabetes.org

AMERICAN DIETETIC ASSOCIATION
120 S. Riverside Plaza, Suite 2000
Chicago, IL 60606
(312) 899-0040
www.eatright.org

ASTHMA/ALLERGY FOUNDATION
OF AMERICA
1125 15th Street, NW, Suite 502
Washington, DC 20005
(800) 7-ASTHMA (help line);
(202) 466-7643 (fax)
www.aafa.org

AUTISM NETWORK-DIET INTERVENTION
(ANDI)
P.O. Box 335
Pennington, NJ 08534
(301) 652-8453 (fax)
www.AutismNDI.com

AUTISM RESEARCH INSTITUTE
5182 Adams Avenue
San Diego, CA 92116
(619) 281-7165; (619) 563-6840 (fax)
www.autismresearchinstitute.com

AUTISM RESOURCE NETWORK
904 Main Street
Hopkins, MN 55343
(952) 988-0088; (952) 988-0099 (fax)
www.autismshop.com

AUTISM SOCIETY OF AMERICA
7910 Woodmont Avenue, Suite 300
Bethesda, MD 20814-3015
(800) 3-Autism, ext. 150 or
(301) 657-0881; (303) 657-0869 (fax)

CELIAC DISEASE CENTER
Columbia University
630 West 168th Street, Box 118
New York, NY 10032
www.celiacdiseasecenter.columbia.edu

CELIAC DISEASE FOUNDATION
13251 Ventura Boulevard, Suite 1
Studio City, CA 91604-1838
(818) 990-2354; (818) 990-2379 (fax)
www.celiac.org/cdf

CELIAC SPRUE ASSOCIATION/USA
P.O. Box 31700
Omaha, NE 68131-0700
877-CSA-4-CSA; (402) 558-1347 (fax)
www.csaceliacs.org

CELIAC SPRUE RESEARCH FOUNDATION
P.O. Box 61193
Palo Alto, CA 94306-1193
www.celiacsupport.stanford.edu

CENTER FOR CELIAC RESEARCH
University of Maryland
20 Penn Street, Room 5303B
Baltimore, MD 21201
www.celiaccenter.org

FEINGOLD ASSOCIATION OF U.S.
P.O. Box 6550
Alexandria, VA 22306
(800) 321-3287
www.feingold.org

FINE, M.D., KENNETH
Intestinal Health Institute
(celiac disease and gluten sensitivity)
www.enterolab.com
www.finerhealth.com

Food Allergy & Anaphylaxis
Network (FAAN)
11781 Lee Jackson Highway, #160
Fairfax, VA 22033
(800) 929-4040 or (703) 691-3179
www.foodallergy.org
fan@worldweb.net
www.fankids.org (for kids)

Friends of Celiac Disease Research
8832 N. Port Washington Road, #204
Milwaukee, WI 53217
(414) 540-6679; (414) 540-0587 (fax)
friends@aero.net

GFCF Diet Support Group
P.O. Box 1692
Palm Harbor, FL 34682
www.gfcfdiet.com

Gluten-Free Living magazine
19A Broadway
Hawthorne, NY 10532
(914) 741-5420
www.glutenfreeliving.com

Gluten Intolerance Group of
North America
15110 10th Avenue SW, Suite A
Seattle, WA 98166-1820
(206) 246-6652; (202) 246-6531 (fax)
www.gluten.net; gig@gluten.net

Living Without magazine
P.O. Box 2126
Northbrook, IL 60065
(847) 480-8810; (847) 480-8810 (fax)
www.livingwithout.com

National Attention Deficit
Disorder Association
1788 Second Street, Suite 200
Highland Park, IL 60035
(847) 432-2332

National Challenged
Homeschoolers Association
Network (N.A.T.H.A.N.)
P.O. Box 39
Porthill, ID 83805
(208) 267-6246
NATHANews@aol.com

National Grain Sorghum
Producers
P.O. Box 5309
Lubbock, TX 79408
(806) 749-3478
www.sorghumgrowers.com

National Jewish Medical
& Research Center
1400 Jackson Street
Denver, CO 80206
(800) 222-5864 (lung line);
(303) 388-4461
www.njc.org

Pathways Medical Advocates
John Hicks, M.D., and Betsy Prohaska Hicks
5411 Highway 50
Delavan, WI 53115
(262) 740-3000
www.pathwaysmed.com

Tri-County Celiac Support Group
47819 Vistas Circle
Canton, MI 48788
gluten-free product list

UNIVERSITY OF CHICAGO CELIAC
DISEASE PROGRAM
5839 S. Maryland Avenue, MC 4065
Chicago, IL 60637-1470
(773) 702-7593; (773) 702-0666 (fax)
http:gi.bsd.uchicago.edu/diseases/
nutritional/celiac_disease.html

YORK NUTRITIONAL LABORATORIES
2700 N. 29th Avenue, Suite 205
Hollywood, FL 33020
(888) 751-3388; (954) 920-3729 (fax)
www.yorkallergyusa.com

ONLINE RESOURCES AND DISCUSSION GROUPS

In addition to the organizations listed on the previous pages, these resources provide additional information and discussions on important topics.

angelfire.com/mi/FAST (articles, recipes, and links)
foodprocessing.com (manufacturer links)
POFAK-subscribe@yahoogroups.com (parents of allergic kids)
www.allergybuyersclub.com (allergy resources, books)
www.allergykids.org/ (allergy kids home page)
www.celiac.com (celiac support page)
www.enabling.org/ia/celiac (celiac disease, gluten sensitivities)
www.fankids.org (Food Allergy Network Web site for kids)
www.funrsc.fairfield.edu/~jfleitas/kidsintro.html ("bandaids and blackboards")
www.glutenfreeinfo.com/Diet/glutenfreeinfo.htm (manufacturer list)
www.nomilk.com (dairy sensitivities)
www.penny.ca/Links.htm (manufacturer links)
www.savorypalate.com (free recipes for gluten sensitivities)
www.yeastconnection.com (the late Dr. William G. Crook's Web site)

INTERNET SUPPORT GROUPS

Celiac Disease, Wheat Sensitivities, and Celiacs with Diabetes
www.enabling.org/ia/celiac/index.html

Dairy Sensitivities: To join, in the body of an e-mail to:
listserv@MAELSTROM.stjohns.edu send the following:

SUB NO-MILK firstname lastname
Also, see www.celiac.com for a wealth of information on the gluten-free diet.

Mail-Order Sources

If you don't have a natural food or specialty food store nearby, the following are mail-order companies that offer gluten-free foods and ingredients. Many also offer products that are free of dairy, eggs, and sugar, but you will need to check each company's Web site for that information. This list is offered as a convenience and is not intended as an endorsement of any particular company nor is it intended to be a complete list of mail-order sources. The names, addresses, phone (or fax) numbers, and e-mail addresses of these companies may have changed as well as the product lines they carry.

AUTHENTIC FOODS
1850 W. 169th Street, Suite B
Gardena, CA 90247
(800) 806-4737; (310) 366-6938 (fax)
www.authenticfoods.com
flours, ingredients, mixes

BOB'S RED MILL NATURAL FOODS
5209 S.E. International Way
Milwaukie, OR 97222
(800) 553-2258; (503) 653-1339 (fax)
www.bobsredmill.com
flours, grains, mixes

CYBROS, INC.
417 Barney Street
Waukesha, WI 53186
(800) 876-2253
bakery items

DIETARY SPECIALTIES
1248 Sussex Turnpike, Unit C-2
Randolph, NJ 07869
(888) 640-2800

www.dietspec.com
foods, ingredients

DOWD & ROGERS
1641 49th Street
Sacramento, CA 95819
(916) 451-6480; (916) 736-2349 (fax)
www.dowdandrogers.com
chestnut flour mixes

ENER-G FOODS, INC.
P.O. Box 84487
Seattle, WA 98124-5787
(800) 331-5222; (206) 764-3398 (fax)
www.ener-g.com
flours, ingredients, mixes

ENJOY LIFE FOODS
1601 Natchez Avenue
Chicago, IL 60707-4023
(888) 50-ENJOY; (773) 889-5090 (fax)
www.enjoylifefoods.com
cookies, bars, bagels, rolled rice flakes

GLUTEN FREE MALL
www.glutenfreemall.com
many vendors offering flours, ingredients,
mixes, food, bakery items, books
(also see www.celiac.com)

GLUTEN FREE MARKET
Route 83 and Lake Cook Road
Buffalo Grove, IL 60089
(847) 419-9610; (847) 419-9615 (fax)
www.glutenfreemarket.com
foods, ingredients, books

GLUTEN-FREE PANTRY
P.O. Box 881
Glastonbury, CT 06033
(203) 633-3826; (860) 633-6853 (fax)
www.glutenfree.com
mixes, ingredients, appliances

GLUTEN-FREE TRADING CO., LLC
604A W. Lincoln Avenue
Milwaukee, WI 53215
(888) 993-9933; (414) 385-9915 (fax)
www.gluten-free.net
flours, ingredients, mixes

GLUTEN SOLUTIONS, INC.
8750 Concourse Court
San Diego, CA 92123
(888) 845-8836; (810) 454-8277 (fax)
www.glutensolutions.com
mixes, ingredients, books, foods

GLUTINO.COM (DEROMA)
1118 Berlier, Laval, Quebec
Canada H7L-3R9
(800) 363-DIET; (450) 629-4781 (fax)
www.glutino.com
mixes, ingredients, baked items

GOODDAY HEALTH
514-A North Western Avenue
Lake Forest, IL 60045
(877) 395-2527; (847) 615-1209 (fax)
gooddayglutenfree@msn.com
gluten-free items, all major vendors

JO'S SPICES (HEALTHY EXCHANGES)
P.O. Box 124, 110 Industrial Street
DeWitt, IA 52742
(319) 659-8234; (319) 659-2126 (fax)
www.healthyexchanges.com
spice blends

KING ARTHUR FLOUR
P.O. Box 876
Norwich, VT 05055-0876
(800) 827-6836; (800) 343-3002 (fax)
www.bakerscatalogue.com
flours, xanthan gum, mixes

KINNIKINNICK FOODS
10940-120 Street
Edmonton, Alberta, Canada, T5H 3P7
(877) 503-4466
www.kinnikinnick.com
flours, baked items, ingredients

MISS ROBEN'S (ALLERGY GROCER)
P.O. Box 1434
Frederick, MD 21702
(800) 891-0083; (301) 631-5954 (fax)
www.missroben.com
baking mixes, ingredients

MONTINA (AMAZING GRAINS)
405 West Main
Ronan, MT 59864
(877) 278-6585; (406) 676-0677 (fax)
www.amazinggrains.com
Indian rice grass flour and mixes

NATURE'S HILIGHTS, INC.
P.O. Box 3526
Chico, CA 95927
(800) 313-6454; (530) 342-3130
www.natures-hilights.com
pizza crusts, snacks, brownies

NUTBALLZ, INC.
1149 Monroe Drive, #B
Boulder, CO 80303
(720) 227-0521; (720) 227-0610 (fax)
www.nutballz.com
gluten-free, sugar-free cookies and bars

NU WORLD AMARANTH
P.O. Box 2202
Naperville, IL 60567
(630) 369-6819
www.nuworldamaranth.com
amaranth flour, amaranth starch, amaranth
snackers, and food products

PAMELA'S PRODUCTS
200 Clara Avenue
Ukiah, CA 95482
(707) 462-6605; (707) 462-6642 (fax)
www.pamelasproducts.com
at gluten-free vendors
cookies, mixes

SHILOH FARMS
Garden Spot Distributors
438 White Oak Road
(800) 829-5100
New Holland, PA 17557
www.gardensspotfinest.com
gluten-free flours, including corn flour

SYLVAN BORDER FARM
P.O. Box 277
Willits, CA 95490-0277
(800) 297-5399; (707) 459-1834 (fax)
www.sylvanborderfarm.com
mixes using quinoa, amaranth, etc.

TRI-COUNTY CELIAC SUPPORT GROUP
47819 Vistas Circle
Canton, MI 48788
gluten-free product list

TWIN VALLEY MILLS, LLC
R.R. 1, Box 45
Ruskin, NE 68974
(402) 279-3965
www.twinvalleymills.com
sorghum flour

VANCE'S FOODS (VANCE'S DARIFREE)
P.O. Box 255734
Sacramento, CA 95865
(800) 497-4834; (800) 497-4329 (fax)
www.vancesfoods.com
dairy-free milk powder and liquid

REFERENCES

Autism Speaks (Autism Coalition for Research and Education). "Autism Facts." www.autismspeaks .org/autism/menu/facts.asp

Braly, James, and Ronald Hoggan. *Dangerous Grains: Why Gluten Cereal Grains May Be Hazardous to Your Health*. New York: Avery, 2002.

Brand-Miller, Jennie, Thomas M. S. Wolever, Kaye Foster-Powell, and Stephen Colagiuri. *The New Glucose Revolution: The Authoritative Guide to the Glycemic Index—the Dietary Solution for Lifelong Health*. New York: Marlowe, 2003.

Brand-Miller, Jennie, Kaye Foster-Powell, Susanna Hold, and Johanna Burani. *The New Glucose Revolution Complete Guide to Glycemic Index Values*. New York: Marlowe, 2003.

Fasano, Alessio, et al. "Prevalence of Celiac Disease in At-Risk and Not-At-Risk Groups in the United States." *Archives of Internal Medicine* 163 (February 10, 2003): 286–92.

Food Allergy & Anaphylaxis Network (FAAN). "Tips for Managing a Milk Allergy." www. food allergy.org/allergens.html#milk

National Institutes of Health (NIH) Consensus Development Conference on Celiac Disease. June 2004. www.consensus.nih.gov/cons/118/118cdc_intro.htm

University of Chicago Celiac Disease Program. "Facts and Figures," 2005. www.uchospitals.edu /specialties/celiac/index.php

University of Maryland Center for Celiac Research. "Legislation Is Passed Making Clearer Food Labels a Reality for Celiac Patients and Allergy Sufferers." www.celiaccenter.org

Whelan, Ann. "Is Vinegar Safe for Celiacs?" *Gluten-Free Living* (September/October 1999): 1, 10, 18.

Whelan, Ann. "Are Natural and Artificial Flavorings Safe?" *Gluten-Free Living* (November/December 1999): 1, 6, 18.

Whelan, Ann. "Don't Worry About Vinegar." *Gluten-Free Living* (Vol. 8, #3): 15–18.

INDEX

About the Author

What began as a solution to Dr. Carol Fenster's own wheat intolerance has grown into an internationally recognized business serving people with food allergies, celiac disease, and autism. Today, Dr. Fenster has published six books and is actively involved and recognized as a leader in the area of food sensitivities. Her books are acknowledged by the Gluten Intolerance Group of North America, the Celiac Disease Foundation, and the Celiac Sprue Association as important resources for celiacs. Many autism organizations also support her work.

Dr. Fenster developed a gluten-free product line for a national company, and she consults with manufacturers and teaches cooking classes. Her recipes appear in numerous books, including those published by the American Dietetic Association. She is a member of the International Association of Culinary Professionals. She appears on *Food for Life,* an allergy-free cooking show on the Health Network. Her articles and recipes and reviews of her books appear in magazines such as *Woman's World, Taste for Life, Vegetarian Times, Veggie Life, Better Nutrition, Gluten-Free Living,* and *Living Without;* professional journals such as *Today's Dietitian;* and newsletters from organizations such as the Food Allergy & Anaphylaxis Network (FAAN), the Gluten Intolerance Group, and the Celiac Disease Foundation. She is the former Associate Food Editor of the magazine *Living Without.*

Dr. Fenster has a degree in home economics from the University of Nebraska. She holds a doctorate in organizational sociology from the University of Denver, where she has also been a faculty member.